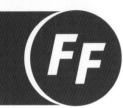

FAST FACTS

*Indispensable
Guides to
Clinical
Practice*

Headach

Second edition

GW00601175

Richard Peatfield

Consultant Neurologist,
West London Neurosciences Centre,
Charing Cross Hospital, London, UK

David W Dodick

Associate Professor,
Mayo Medical School;
Consultant Neurologist,
Department of Neurology,
Mayo Clinic, Scottsdale,
Arizona, USA

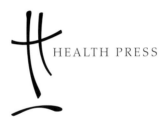

HEALTH PRESS

Oxford

Fast Facts – Headaches
First published 2000
Second edition December 2002

Text © 2002 Richard Peatfield, David W Dodick
© 2002 in this edition Health Press Limited
Health Press Limited, Elizabeth House, Queen Street,
Abingdon, Oxford OX14 3JR, UK
Tel: +44 (0)1235 523233
Fax: +44 (0)1235 523238

Fast Facts is a trade mark of Health Press Limited.

A CIP catalogue record for this title is available from the British Library.

ISBN 1-903734-21-5

Peatfield, R (Richard)
Fast Facts – Headaches/
Richard Peatfield, David W Dodick

Typeset by Zed, Oxford, UK

Printed by Fine Print (Services) Ltd, Oxford, UK.

Glossary

Arnold–Chiari malformation: a congenital disorder in which the base of the brain is distorted and the lower brainstem and part of the cerebellum protrude through the opening at the base of the skull

Aura: a premonitory, subjective sensation preceding an attack of migraine or epilepsy

AVM: arteriovenous malformation. Cluster of distended blood vessels that press on the brain

BIH: benign intracranial hypertension

CADASIL: cerebral autosomal-dominant arteriopathy with subcortical infarcts and leukoencephalopathy

CBF: cerebral blood flow

CDH: chronic daily headache

CGRP: calcitonin gene-related peptide

CH: cluster headache

CSF: cerebrospinal fluid

CT: computed tomography, a radiological method of imaging soft tissues

CVST: cerebral venous sinus thrombosis

Diplopia: double vision

Hemianopia: condition where half the normal field of vision is absent

Horner's syndrome: drooping of an upper eyelid, constriction of the pupil, and an absence of sweating over the affected side of the face. The syndrome is caused by a nervous disorder in the brainstem or neck

IHS: International Headache Society

5-HT: 5-hydroxytryptamine or serotonin, a widely distributed biochemical that may play a role in the modulation of craniovascular pain

MRI: magnetic resonance imaging, a non-radiological method of obtaining a cross-sectional image of tissues and systems

Neuralgia: a painful affection of the nerves

NO: nitric oxide, an endogenous mediator of physiological vasodilation

NSAIDs: non-steroidal anti-inflammatory drugs, commonly used for analgesia in headache

Papilledema: swelling of the first portion of the optic nerve

PET: positron emission tomography, a method of imaging to determine the metabolic activity of various regions of the brain

SAH: subarachnoid hemorrhage

SUNCT: short-lasting unilateral neuralgiform pain with conjuctival injection and tearing

Scotoma (plural scotomata): a small area in the visual field where vision is absent

Serotonin: *see* 5-HT

TTH: tension-type headache

Vasodilator: a nerve or agent bringing about vasodilation of blood vessels

Introduction

Most people experience at least occasional headaches during their lifetime. Although many sufferers can function normally using self-medication, the management of patients with disabling headaches forms a substantial proportion of the workload for family physicians and practicing neurologists. In a small number of patients, headache is a symptom of a potentially serious illness, and the first task of any physician is to identify and treat these conditions. Most patients seek reassurance that their headache is benign and that self-medication is appropriate. Many of these people experience disabling headaches, either continuously or as attacks, that justify careful assessment and specific intermittent or regular therapies available only on prescription.

This book describes the processes used to assess patients with headache, summarizes current thinking on pathogenesis and outlines the management of the common forms of disabling primary headache. Most assessment and treatment can, and indeed should, be undertaken within the primary care setting; only patients who are severely affected or refractory to treatment require specialist referral for investigation. The reassurance of people who are healthy but worried, and the proper investigation and treatment of those who are unwell are vital components of the role of any physician, and are particularly rewarding in patients with headache.

A positive diagnosis must be made at or soon after the first consultation with a patient seeking advice about headache. Most patients, especially with primary headache disorders, have few, if any, physical abnormalities to provide clinical clues, so the assessment must be derived largely from clinical history. A physical examination seldom provides much information, and special investigations are useful only in excluding specific structural secondary causes for headaches. It is, therefore, essential for both the family physician and the specialist to document the patient's complaint carefully, as this will usually be the sole basis on which the working clinical diagnosis can be made.

The clinician should record:
- the duration of headache
- the pattern of attacks, with their duration, severity and frequency
- the presence or absence of accompanying symptoms, such as nausea or vomiting, or visual, limb or speech disturbances.

The relationship of headache to coughing, foods, exercise, and neck and jaw movements may also be significant.

The majority of patients seen in the primary care setting have tension-type or migraine headache (Table 1.1); most recurrent, severe headaches are migrainous and are more likely to need to be referred on for specialist assessment and advice. In general, patients with recurrent non-progressive headache without significant disability or physical abnormalities should be reassured by the family physician and offered migraine-specific medication or appropriately potent analgesics, since the majority will have tried simple, non-prescription analgesics prior to seeking medical attention. In contrast, patients with any of the characteristics listed in Table 1.2 should be considered for referral for specialist care.

Secondary causes of headache (e.g. cervical spondylosis, post-traumatic headache and sinusitis) and headache associated with febrile illnesses, such as influenza, are responsible for no more than 5% of cases referred to a neurological outpatient clinic. Intracranial space-

TABLE 1.1

Differential diagnosis of headache

Primary

- Migraine*
  - episodic
  - chronic

- Tension-type headache*
  - episodic
  - chronic

- Cluster headache*
  - episodic
  - chronic

- Benign exertional headache

Secondary

- Cerebral tumors

- Hydrocephalus and CSF obstruction

- Low-pressure headache

- Spontaneous intracranial hypotension

- Arteriovenous malformations

- Cervicogenic headache

- Sinusitis

- Temporal arteritis

- Meningitis/encephalitis

- Subarachnoid hemorrhage

- Hypertension

- Cerebrovascular disease
  - transient ischemic attacks
  - stroke
  - carotid endarterectomy
  - cerebral venous sinus thrombosis
  - arterial dissection

- Cranial neuralgias
  - trigeminal
  - post-herpetic

- Facial and dental pain

- Analgesia-induced headaches

- Post-traumatic headaches

- Other benign headaches*
  - drug-induced headache
  - food- and alcohol-induced headache

* Discussed in other chapters

occupying lesions, such as gliomas, meningiomas, cerebral abscesses and hematomas, are unusual in an outpatient setting. Although the majority of patients seen in a hospital emergency department complaining of 'the worst headache of my life' are still more likely to have a primary headache disorder, a higher proportion than in an

TABLE 1.2

Characteristics of patients requiring further investigation and referral

- Suspected recent subarachnoid hemorrhage or meningitis
- Abnormal neurological physical signs (e.g. papilledema, hemiparesis, permanent visual loss and ataxia)
- Decrease in visual acuity or temporary loss of vision
- Persistent or increasing vomiting
- Headache of recent onset or increasing frequency or severity
- Seizures
- Endocrine disturbances (e.g. acromegaly, diabetes insipidus, amenorrhea, galactorrhea, impaired male sexual function or beard growth and poor growth in children)
- Relevant past or family history, such as previous malignancies or neurofibromatosis

outpatient clinic have a secondary headache, particularly sinusitis, subarachnoid hemorrhage or meningitis (Figure 1.1). New-onset headache or a change from a previous pattern should, therefore, always prompt neuroimaging and/or CSF studies before it is deemed primary.

Cerebral tumors

Headache is a common symptom of space-occupying intracranial lesions, such as:
- primary brain tumors
- cerebral metastases
- other masses, including subdural hematomas and cerebral abscesses.

The presence of headache becomes more likely as the tumor expands, and is almost universal in the terminal stages. Headache is seldom the only reason why a patient with a cerebral tumor seeks advice. Most patients present with either seizures or a focal cerebral dysfunction reflecting tumor invasion, rather than distortion of intracranial structures (Figure 1.2). Investigations should be directed at the cause of these symptoms or signs, as the reason for the headache then often becomes evident.

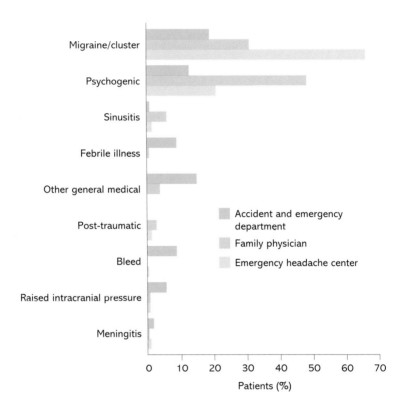

Figure 1.1 Cause/type of headache in patients attending an accident and emergency department, their family physician, or an emergency headache center. Data from Fodden et al. 1989, Bass et al. 1996, and Ducros et al. 2001.

Patients giving a history of subacute headache, especially if associated with seizures or abnormal physical findings, warrant urgent investigation. However, surveys of patients with proven tumors support the view that the proportion without these clues is so small that routine scanning is uneconomical. In most cases, reviewing the patient after 3 months will establish that the headache pattern is, indeed, benign.

Routine computed tomography (CT) scanning fails to detect many cases of Arnold–Chiari malformations, meningitis, carotid/vertebral dissection, cerebral venous sinus thrombosis, high-/low-pressure syndromes, giant-cell arteritis and leptomeningeal disease. Therefore, a

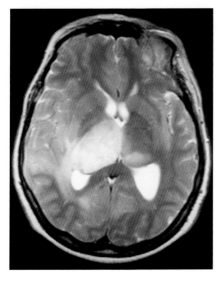

Figure 1.2 MRI scan of a 60-year-old woman who was referred to the migraine clinic with a 3-month history of right temporoparietal headaches with fortification phenomena in the right field of vision. Six weeks later, before she could be seen, she had three focal seizures involving the left arm and leg. There were no signs, but CT and MRI scans showed a mass lesion which was found to be a grade II glioma after stereotactic biopsy.

normal scan does not necessarily mean that a patient has a benign migraine-like headache if the results of careful clinical assessment indicate otherwise.

Hydrocephalus and cerebrospinal fluid obstruction

Headache is an uncommon symptom in long-standing obstructive or 'normal pressure'-type hydrocephalus. It is, however, often found in acute obstructions of CSF pathways due to cerebral tumors at any site (particularly in the posterior fossa) or to obstructive lesions within the ventricular system, such as colloid cysts of the third ventricle, when it can be triggered by changes in position. Most of these patients have papilledema, and a scan can establish its cause. Definitive surgical treatment is necessary in the majority of theses cases.

All headaches may be worsened by coughing, straining, sneezing or bending over. However, those triggered de novo by a cough or other maneuver that raises intracranial pressure may be caused by an obstruction of the ventricular system – either a major posterior fossa tumor or an Arnold–Chiari malformation in which the cerebellar tonsils block the foramen magnum. The presence of an Arnold–Chiari malformation is best confirmed by a sagittal magnetic resonance imaging (MRI) scan (Figure 1.3). The obstruction may be relieved by surgical decompression of the foramen magnum, usually with relief of the cough headache.

Benign intracranial hypertension

Some patients, often women, presenting with rapidly progressive headache and papilledema may be found on scanning to have small, slit-like ventricles, suggesting generalized swelling of the brain substance rather than ventricle enlargement or an intracranial mass. Some of these patients describe blurred or obscured vision symptomatic of papilledema, nausea with or without vomiting, or diplopia usually due to sixth nerve palsy. Lumbar puncture is usually considered safe as long as the patient remains fully conscious. This will reveal a raised CSF pressure, which is often above 200 mmCSF.

The cause of the raised intracranial pressure is not clearly established. Patients with cerebral venous sinus thrombosis (CVST) commonly present with this clinical picture. The thrombosis is usually evident on MRI scans (or MR venography) and can be confirmed angiographically. Since 25% of patients with suspected BIH (pseudotumor) have CVST, many authorities recommend routine angiography or magnetic resonance venography in people with BIH. Other cases of BIH are associated with head injuries, tetracycline or initiation or withdrawal of corticosteroids.

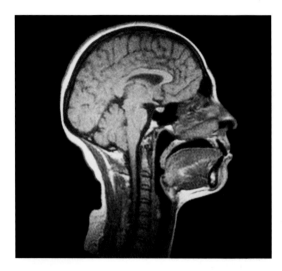

Figure 1.3 Sagittal MRI scan of a woman with cough headache showing an Arnold–Chiari malformation.

Many patients with the condition are significantly obese and improve after weight reduction. The headache is often relieved by CSF removal at the original lumbar puncture. Acetazolamide and other diuretics are often used to reduce the rate of CSF production. Headaches that persist and threaten the patient's vision can often be relieved by insertion of a lumboperitoneal shunt or by an optic nerve sheath fenestration.

Low-pressure headache

About one-third of people experience headache following lumbar puncture. This headache is made worse if the patient sits up, is relieved by lying down and usually fades within a few days. It is believed to be due to leakage of spinal fluid through the hole in the dura. Other patients experience similar headaches without a clear-cut cause, which are sometimes found to be due to a spontaneous dural tear. The dura often enhance with gadolinium on MRI scanning (Figure 1.4), though the mechanism of this is uncertain. Most low-pressure headaches resolve spontaneously, but the process can be accelerated by an epidural blood patch even if it is not over the site of the presumed leak. A few patients, however, require direct surgical repair of the dural defect (Figure 1.5).

Arteriovenous malformations

Knotted masses of distended blood vessels forming high-flow, fistulous communications between arteries and veins may occur in all parts of the brain. These produce a typical area on a CT or MRI scan enhanced with intravenous contrast, usually without distortion of adjacent structures. The size of these malformations and the nature of their blood supply vessel can be confirmed by arteriography if appropriate. Many come to medical attention by rupturing into the brain substance or subarachnoid space, and a few cause epilepsy. They occasionally cause headaches resembling migraine, and large surveys have shown an increased prevalence of malformations among migrainous patients. Recognized treatments for the malformations include direct surgical excision, embolization via an intra-arterial catheter and localized radiotherapy. These interventions carry risks that may be justified in

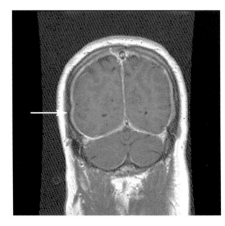

Figure 1.4 T1 weighted coronal MRI with contrast in a patient with spontaneous intracranial hypotension secondary to a spontaneous CSF leak. Note the pachymeningeal thickening and enhancement.

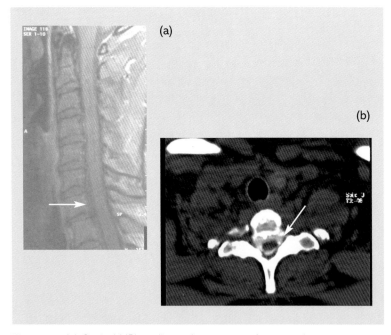

(a)

(b)

Figure 1.5 (a) Sagittal MRI gradient echo sequence demonstrating extra-arachnoid CSF collection (arrow) anterior to the spinal cord at C5–T2. (b) CT/myelogram demonstrates CSF collection (arrow) with a disk/osteophyte complex protruding into it. At surgery, this 38-year-old woman was found to have a disk adhering to the dura at C6, with a tear in the dura and penetration by the disk. The dural tear was repaired, the CSF leak occluded, and the patient became headache-free.

patients whose malformations have already bled, but are probably not justified in those complaining only of headache.

Cervicogenic headache

Radiological evidence of cervical spondylosis is found almost universally in elderly people. Some patients complain of pain not only in the neck but also radiating forwards beyond the vertex towards the forehead, and probably related to an overlap with trigeminal relays in the brainstem (Figure 1.6). This pain is usually constant and can be unilateral, and is worsened by neck movements. Physical examination demonstrates restricted mobility, particularly of lateral flexion, without any other abnormalities; it is always prudent to carry out an

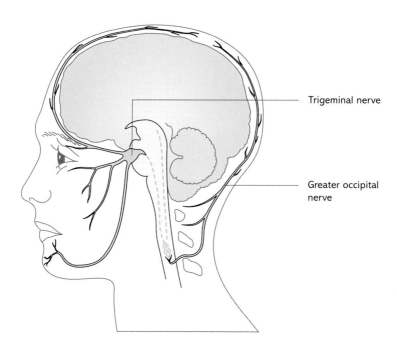

Trigeminal nerve

Greater occipital nerve

Figure 1.6 Trigeminal connections within the brainstem. Adapted with permission from Lance. *Mechanism and Management of Headache*. 4th edn. London: Butterworth & Co., 1982.

erythrocyte sedimentation rate (ESR) test to exclude temporal arteritis in older patients with headache of recent onset. Physical therapy, local massage and simple analgesics or NSAIDs may be helpful. In treatment-resistant patients with severe pain/headaches, relief may be obtained by blockade of the greater occipital nerve or C2 facet with corticosteroid and local anesthesia.

Sinusitis

Sinusitic pain is commonly seen in primary care and emergency department settings, and is unusual in a neurological clinic. Most patients report that their pain started after a recent upper respiratory tract infection, and is associated with malaise, pyrexia, facial tenderness and a purulent discharge from the nose or into the nasopharynx. The pain may be referred to the forehead, temples or vertex depending on the sinus or sinuses involved. Maxillary sinusitis causes deep central face pain. Pain from the frontal sinuses usually starts an hour or two after rising, clearing up in the afternoon, while that from the maxillary sinuses is worse on waking and is relieved by getting up. Malignant disease of the sinuses should not be overlooked as a cause of chronic discomfort associated with radiological opacification of the sinuses. Sinusitis, however, is generally not a cause of recurrent severe headaches – many patients with migraine are mistakenly diagnosed with 'sinus headache'.

Temporal arteritis

Temporal or giant-cell arteritis seldom occurs in people under 55 years of age, but becomes progressively more common in each subsequent decade. The pain is not always confined to one temple and may be frontal, occipital or more generalized. All elderly patients with a recent history of headache should have their ESR and/or C-reactive protein level checked with this diagnosis in mind. It may be appropriate to arrange a temporal artery biopsy in patients with an otherwise unexplained elevated ESR, and in those with a typical history. Any patient suspected of having temporal arteritis should be given high-dose steroids (e.g. prednisone, 80 mg/day) at once; biopsy changes take several days to begin to resolve, and the diagnosis is strongly supported by an overnight response to high-dose steroids. The prednisone dose can then be tapered down gradually over 1–2 years, ensuring that the ESR remains within normal limits. Temporal arteritis is not adequately controlled by alternate-day steroid regimens, and steroid-induced complications (most commonly osteoporotic vertebral collapse) are occasionally seen despite the use of the lowest dose sufficient to control the ESR and headache.

Meningitis/encephalitis

Acute meningitis is rarely found in a neurological outpatient setting and is almost as unusual in routine primary care, but it is commonly seen in emergency situations. Most patients with meningitis have pyrexia and neck stiffness or a positive Kernig's sign, though tuberculous meningitis may develop more insidiously. Broad-spectrum conventional antibiotics should be administered once meningitis is suspected; this treatment will cause no harm if the headache is later shown to be viral in origin or due to a subarachnoid hemorrhage.

The diagnosis is confirmed by lumbar puncture, which is usually best carried out after scanning. The CSF will contain neutrophils or lymphocytes, with a low glucose level in bacterial or fungal disease but not in viral meningitis. It is important to be aware of the possibility of insidious meningeal infections, particularly in debilitated or immunosuppressed patients, including those with AIDS. These include tuberculous meningitis and sarcoidosis, cryptococcal and other fungal infections, Behçet's syndrome and Lyme disease.

Subarachnoid hemorrhage

Subarachnoid hemorrhage (SAH) due to a ruptured arterial aneurysm or arteriovenous malformation (AVM) almost always causes a headache of devastatingly sudden onset, in which loss of consciousness and sudden death are common. Headache may be the sole manifestation in approximately 12% of patients with SAH. In patients able to complain of headache, the suddenness of onset is the most important clue, as neck stiffness, if it occurs, may take up to 3 hours to develop.

Urgent referral is essential for patients in whom SAH is suspected. CT scanning has been found to be diagnostic in 98% within the first

12 hours after the onset of headache, falling to 93% by 24 hours. Expert neuroradiologists, however, interpreted the CT scans in most of these studies, and other physicians less experienced in reading CT scans may overlook subtle abnormalities. Furthermore, the sensitivity of CT scanning decreases to 76% 2 days after the onset of headache, and to 58% 5 days later.

A lumbar puncture therefore is required in all patients whose initial CT scan is negative, equivocal or technically inadequate. The CSF pressure should always be measured, as high intracranial pressure may be an important clue to the presence of an active intracranial event such as SAH or CVST. Elevated opening pressure may also help distinguish between a traumatic lumbar puncture and a subarachnoid hemorrhage. It is vital that this distinction be made since about 20% of lumbar punctures are traumatic, and simply observing for a decrement in the erythrocyte count in three successive tubes is not entirely reliable. In addition, if the fluid is not promptly centrifuged and examined, erythrocytes resulting from a traumatic tap may undergo lysis in vitro, producing xanthochromia from the formation of oxyhemoglobin. Visual inspection for xanthochromia can miss discoloration in up to 50% of specimens. The detection of xanthochromia by spectrophotometry is the most accurate test for subarachnoid hemorrhage, with a sensitivity of 100% when a lumbar puncture is performed between 12 hours and 2 weeks after the ictus.

Although thunderclap headache, an excruciating headache of instantaneous onset, is the sine qua non of subarachnoid hemorrhage, in some patients there may be no underlying secondary cause, while in others transient diffuse vasospasm in the absence of subarachnoid hemorrhage is detected on angiography. Although idiopathic thunderclap headache may represent a distinct primary headache syndrome, an indistinguishable headache profile may occur in the setting of sinister intracranial and extracranial vascular pathology. Similar sudden peak-intensity headaches with normal neurological examinations can be the presenting feature of CVST, pituitary apoplexy, arterial dissection, acute hypertensive crisis, spontaneous retroclival hematomas, and spontaneous intracranial hypotension. These disorders, with the exception of subarachnoid hemorrhage, may evade detection by CT and lumbar puncture. Careful clinical assessment and appropriate MRI are crucial in diagnosing these disorders.

Hypertension

When hypertension is so severe that patients develop features such as papilledema, it is often associated with headache. However, more modest elevations of blood pressure that justify treatment do not usually cause headache, and head pain usually has a different cause. Vasodilators given for hypertension, particularly nifedipine, hydralazine and reserpine, are potent causes of headache, though β-blockers may relieve the pain. In contrast, sudden rises in blood pressure due to a pheochromocytoma often cause paroxysms of headache, and occasional patients with such attacks should be investigated with this diagnosis in mind.

Cerebrovascular disease

Transient ischemic attacks. Headache occurs in 6–44% of patients with transient ischemic attacks. If ischemia is in the carotid territory the headache is usually perceived in the frontal region, and it is occipital if the patient has a vertebrobasilar embolism. The pain is usually mild to moderate in severity, usually on the same side as the vascular disturbance, and lasts for a few hours. It may be difficult to distinguish this headache from that induced by a small subarachnoid hemorrhage, and a lumbar puncture is sometimes justified.

Stroke. Headache is a common feature of stroke. It is seen in 20–30% of patients with large artery occlusions, though it is unusual in lacunar infarction. The mechanism of this headache is uncertain; it may relate to dilation of collateral vessels or the release of mediators from vessel walls. Again, the headache is usually ipsilateral to the hemisphere disturbance, but its duration is variable.

Carotid endarterectomy. Headache is commonly seen after carotid endarterectomy. It is usually ipsilateral to the location of the procedure and may develop some hours after it. Although the etiology is unclear, surgical interference with the sympathetic nervous supply running along the arterial wall at the site of the operation, or sudden reperfusion of distal vessels, are possible mechanisms.

Cerebral venous sinus thrombosis. Headache is the most common symptom of CVST, occurring in about 75% of cases. It may be diffuse or localized, and it is most often persistent, worse upon recumbency, and aggravated by a Valsalva maneuver. Although its onset is usually subacute over several days, up to 10% of patients with CVST may present with thunderclap headache. Overall, CT scans are interpreted as normal in about 25% of patients with CVST. This proportion reaches 50% or more in patients with isolated intracranial hypertension but is below 10% in patients with focal neurological signs. Although the CSF is abnormal in 30–50% of published cases, with some combination of lymphocytic pleocytosis, red blood cells and elevated protein, up to 40% of patients with CVST may have an elevated opening pressure with otherwise normal CSF. When there is a clinical suspicion of CVST, a MRI scan should be the initial investigation (Figure 1.7).

Carotid artery dissection. Headache is also the earliest and most common clinical manifestation of symptomatic internal carotid artery dissection, occurring in up to 75% of patients. Usually there is oculosympathetic paresis (Horner's syndrome) and a unilateral frontal headache; however, delayed focal cerebral ischemic events are also a common presentation. The headache can be instantaneous and severe.

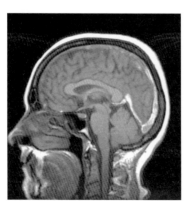

Figure 1.7 Sagittal T1-weighted MRI scan of brain demonstrating acute thrombosis of the straight and sagittal sinus.

Unless the arterial dissection is accompanied by ischemic stroke, CT scanning and lumbar puncture are unhelpful; MR angiography is fast becoming the test of choice to demonstrate the dissection. The outcome of internal carotid artery dissection is generally favorable, but permanent neurological deficits and even death may result from acute ischemic stroke. Although no controlled trials are available, early identification of arterial dissection may allow early initiation of antiplatelet or anticoagulation therapy, possibly preventing more serious cerebral ischemic complications.

Cranial neuralgias

Trigeminal neuralgia. The pain of trigeminal neuralgia usually affects the mandibular or maxillary divisions of the trigeminal nerve on one side. The patient experiences very severe 'lancinating' pains lasting for only seconds and is pain-free between them. The pains are often triggered by innocuous local stimuli, such as eating, touching the face or even gusts of wind. In most cases, the pain is believed to be due to an elongated or ectatic artery in the posterior fossa impinging on the trigeminal nerve as it enters the pons, though in a small number of patients under 50 years it is a symptom of a multiple sclerosis plaque within the brainstem. Neuralgias are best managed with anticonvulsants, including carbamazepine, oxcarbazepine or gabapentin. A variety of surgical and radiation treatments are available for patients with refractory neuralgia. These include: percutaneous neurolytic procedures targeting the trigeminal ganglion; posterior fossa microvascular decompression; and gamma knife radiosurgery targeting the trigeminal root entry zone near the brainstem.

An analogous symptom is seen when the ninth cranial nerve is affected, in which pain usually radiates from the tonsillar fossa to the ear or angle of the mandible and is triggered by swallowing.

Post-herpetic neuralgia. Persistent, deep-seated pain of a different character may follow focal herpes zoster infection in the trigeminal distribution, particularly in older patients (over 70 years). The pain may be a dull ache of great severity, and is thought to be due to destruction of the larger nerve fibers supplying the dermatome. Its management is often difficult. Attempts to increase the non-noxious sensory input in adjacent segments with cold or vibrating stimuli may be of value, and tricyclic antidepressants, anticonvulsants, topical anesthetics, or combinations of these agents have also shown benefits.

Facial and dental pain

It is usually easy to identify pain caused by disease of the teeth or temporo-mandibular joint, as this is usually localized and increased by jaw movements. Once trigeminal neuralgia, cluster headache and diseases of the teeth, ears, eyes and related structures have been excluded, most patients with unilateral facial pain will have a disorder classified as 'atypical facial pain'. These patients usually respond to antidepressants even if they are not overtly depressed.

Other benign headaches

Exertional headaches. At least three mechanisms cause headache triggered by exertion:

- surge in blood pressure
- Valsalva's maneuver, inhibiting venous drainage from the brain and thus increasing intracranial pressure
- hyperdynamic circulation.

Weightlifter's headache is probably precipitated by a Valsalva's maneuver, whereas runner's headache may be due to hyperdynamic circulation.

Benign coital headache probably involves a combination of all three mechanisms. It is a 'capricious' phenomenon that often occurs several times, though patients need to be reassured that it need not occur on every occasion. A single episode of headache arising during sexual intercourse must be investigated as a possible subarachnoid hemorrhage.

Many patients with benign exertional headache respond to either propranolol or indomethacin, either given regularly or to pre-empt a particular triggering situation.

Drug-induced headache. The headache induced by vasodilators has already been mentioned (see page 19). Headache induced by the regular consumption of ergotamine or codeine-containing analgesics is described in Chapter 6. Glyceryl trinitrate, indomethacin and dipyridamole are also common causes of headache. The contraceptive pill may also cause headache (see Chapter 5).

Headache induced by food and ethanol. The role of foods in precipitating migrainous headache is discussed in Chapter 5. A number of food additives, including nitrites, the sweetener aspartame and monosodium glutamate ('Chinese restaurant syndrome'), warrant a mention. The mechanism of hangover is complex and poorly understood; in most patients, the principal symptom is a throbbing headache, which can last for many hours and is worsened by head movements. Tremor, nervousness, depression, flushes, and nausea and vomiting are symptoms described as 'hangover' by alcoholics, but these may be mediated differently. The symptoms of a hangover appear long after all alcohol has been metabolized. Possible mechanisms include dehydration due to the alcohol's diuretic effect, a toxic effect of acetaldehyde (common in Oriental people), hepatic dysfunction and disruption of sleep. Hypoglycemia is regarded as unimportant.

Differential diagnosis – Key points

- Most recurring headaches are benign.
- Very few patients with tumors present with headaches; those with headache for longer than 3 months, and with no focal symptoms or physical signs, do not normally need investigation.
- Subarachnoid hemorrhage must be excluded in patients presenting with headache of sudden onset.
- Cervical spondylosis is the commonest cause of *new* headache in older people, but always think of temporal arteritis.
- New headache in a sick, febrile patient might be due to meningitis; it is advisable to give antibiotics first, and investigate later.

Key references

General reference works and reviews

Fodden DI, Peatfield RC, Milsom PL. Beware the patient with a headache in the accident and emergency department. *Arch Emergency Med* 1989;6:7–12.

Goadsby PJ, Lipton RB, Ferrari MD. Drug therapy: migraine – current understanding and treatment. *N Engl J Med* 2002;346:257–70.

Olesen J, Tfelt-Hansen P, Welch KMA, eds. *The Headaches*, 2nd edn. New York: Raven Press, 1999.

Peatfield RC, Fozard JR, Clifford Rose F. Drug treatment of migraine. In: *Handbook of Clinical Neurology*. Amsterdam: Elsevier, 1986:173–216.

Sandler M, Ferrari M, Harnett S. *Migraine: Pharmacology and Genetics*. London: Altman, 1996.

Silberstein S, Goadsby PJ, Lipton RB. *Headache in Clinical Practice*. Oxford: Isis Medical, 1998.

Sjaastad O. *Cluster Headache Syndrome*. London: WB Saunders, 1992.

Primary literature

Bass MH, McWhinney IR, Dempsey JB et al. Predictors of outcomes in headache patients presenting to family physicians – a one-year prospective study. *Headache* 1986;26:285–94.

Ducros A, El Amrani M, Slamia LB et al. The first 3 months of the Lariboisiere Emergency Headache Center: a series of 3799 patients. *Cephalalgia* 2001;21:322.

Edlow JA, Caplan LR. Avoiding pitfalls in the diagnosis of subarachnoid hemorrhage. *N Engl J Med* 2000;342(1):29–36.

Frishberg BM. The utility of neuroimaging in the evaluation of headache in patients with normal neurologic examinations. *Neurology* 1994;44:1191–7.

Lance JW. Headaches related to sexual activity. *J Neurol Neurosurg Psychiatry* 1976;39:1226–30.

Marcelis J, Silberstein SD. Idiopathic intracranial hypertension without papilloedema. *Arch Neurol* 1991;48:392–9.

Mason JC, Walport MJ. Giant cell arteritis. *BMJ* 1992;305:68–9.

Nightingale S, Williams B. Hindbrain hernia headache. *Lancet* 1987;1:731–4.

Ostergaard JR. Warning leak in subarachnoid haemorrhage. *BMJ* 1990;301:190–1.

Walchenbach R, Voormolen JHC. Surgical treatment for trigeminal neuralgia. *BMJ* 1996;313:1027–8.

Wijdicks EFM, Kerkhoff H, Van Gijn J. Long-term follow-up of 71 patients with thunderclap headache mimicking subarachnoid haemorrhage. *Lancet* 1988;2:68–70.

Headache is a subjective symptom which may be part of a complex primary disorder such as migraine or a manifestation of an underlying disease process. Like any symptom for which there are no objective markers, an accurate classification system is essential for accurate diagnosis and appropriate treatment. In 1988 the International Headache Society instituted a classification system which established uniform terminology and consistent diagnostic criteria for a range of headache disorders (see, for example, Tables 2.1 and 2.2). This system has become the standard for headache diagnosis, endorsed by the World Health Organization and incorporated into the International Classification of Diseases (ICD-10). It has facilitated epidemiological research and clinical drug trials across the world and provides the basis for current research and treatment guidelines.

These definitions have been used by Rasmussen and the Copenhagen group to obtain prevalence figures for migraine and tension headache (Figure 2.1). The results of comparable studies have been reported from Denmark, France, Canada, Germany and the USA (Table 2.3).

Two methodologically identical national surveys in the USA conducted 10 years apart recently showed that the prevalence and distribution of migraine have remained stable over the last decade, and that migraine-associated disability remains substantial and pervasive. The number of migraineurs increased from 23.6 million in 1989 to 27.9 million in 1999, commensurate with the growth of the population. The prevalence of migraine was 18.2% among females and 6.5% among males. Approximately 23% of households contained at least one member suffering from migraine. Migraine prevalence was higher in whites than in blacks and was inversely related to household income. Prevalence increased from age 12 years to about age 40 years and declined thereafter in both sexes. Fifty-three percent of respondents reported that their severe headaches caused substantial impairment in activities or required bed rest. Approximately 31% had missed at least 1 day of work or school in the previous 3 months because of migraine,

TABLE 2.1

International Headache Society diagnostic criteria for migraine

Migraine

Migraine without aura

A At least five attacks fulfilling B–D

B Headache attacks lasting 4–72 hours (untreated or unsuccessfully treated)

C Headache has at least two of the following characteristics:

1 Unilateral location

2 Pulsating quality

3 Moderate or severe intensity

4 Aggravation by walking on stairs or similar routine physical activity

D During headache, at least one of the following:

1 Nausea and/or vomiting

2 Photophobia and phonophobia

Migraine with aura

A At least two attacks fulfilling B

B At least three of the following characteristics:

1 One or more fully reversible aura symptoms indicating focal cerebral cortical and/or brainstem dysfunction

2 At least one aura symptom develops gradually over more than 4 minutes, or two or more symptoms occur in succession

3 No aura symptom lasts for more than 60 minutes. If more than one aura symptom is present, accepted duration is proportionally increased

4 Headache follows aura with a free interval of less than 60 minutes (it may also begin before or simultaneously with the aura)

TABLE 2.2

International Headache Society diagnostic criteria for tension-type headache

A	At least 10 attacks fulfilling B–D
B	Headache lasting from 30 min to 7 days
C	At least 2 of the following pain characteristics: 1 Non-pulsating quality 2 Mild to moderate intensity (may inhibit, but does not prohibit activities) 3 Bilateral location 4 No aggravation on exercise
D	Both of the following: 1 No nausea or vomiting 2 No more than one of photophobia and phonophobia

Reproduced, with permission, from Headache Classification Committee of the International Headache Society 1988

while 51% reported that work or school productivity was reduced by at least 50%. Migraine is therefore a major cause of absenteeism from and decreased productivity at work, demonstrably reduces health-related quality of life, and costs American employers approximately $13 billion per year.

Genetics of migraine

Most people seeking advice about migraine have relatives who are also affected. If there is a genetic component to migraine, first-degree relatives of patients will have a substantially higher risk of having migraine than members of the population as a whole. Epidemiological studies undertaken in Copenhagen showed that the relative risk of having migraine without aura in first-degree relatives of patients with migraine without aura was 1.9, with a relative risk of 1.4 for migraine with aura. If the index patient had migraine with aura there was no

27

increased risk of migraine without aura, but migraine with aura was 3.8 times more likely to occur. These findings suggest that additional genetic factors may contribute only to migraine with aura.

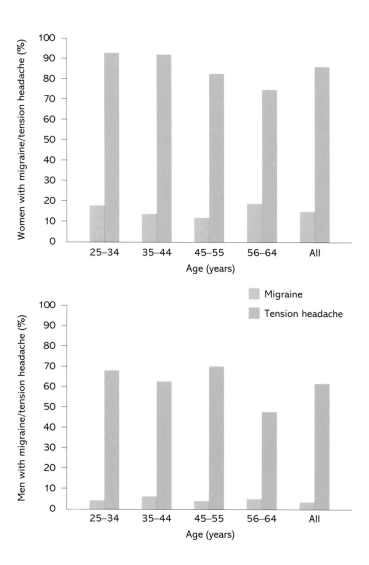

Figure 2.1 Prevalence of migraine and tension headache in a study of 387 men and 353 women (1-year prevalence on 23 November 1988). Data from Rasmussen et al. 1991.

TABLE 2.3

Studies of 1-year prevalence of migraine using the International
Headache Society classification*

Age range studied (years)	Sample size (n)	Methodology	Males with migraine (%)	Females with migraine (%)	Reference
Denmark					
25–64	740	Random sample of suburban population	5.9	15.3	Rasmussen et al. 1991
France					
> 15	4204	Nationwide representative sample	6.1	17.6	Henry et al. 1992
USA					
21–30	1007	Health maintenance organization	3.4	12.9	Breslau et al. 1991
12–80	20468	Representative households	5.7	17.6	Stewart et al. 1992
Canada					
> 18	2292	Randomly telephoned households	7.4	21.9	O'Brien et al. 1994
Germany					
> 18	4061	Mailing to stratified households	7.0	15.0	Göbel et al. 1994

*Reproduced with permission from *Current Medical Literature (Neurology)* 1996;12:60

Comparisons of migraine prevalence in monozygotic and dizygotic twins suggest that 40–50% of the tendency to develop migraine is attributable to genetic factors. It is likely that a small number of separate genes contribute to migraine, some of which are involved in the development of aura symptoms.

Familial hemiplegic migraine is the only variety of migraine in which a Mendelian type of inheritance has been clearly established. This rare variety of migraine with aura is characterized by an autosomal-dominant pattern of inheritance, by the presence of hemiparesis during attacks, and, in some patients, severe coma with prolonged hemiplegia. Some patients have permanent neurological signs such as nystagmus and ataxia between attacks. Some families with the condition have a defect on chromosome 19 that codes for the α_{1A} subunit of a calcium channel; others map to chromosome 1, and some cannot so far be located. There is also evidence that this calcium channel gene on chromosome 19 is linked to more common varieties of migraine.

Migraine also presents with an autosomal-dominant pattern in some families with cerebral autosomal-dominant arteriopathy with

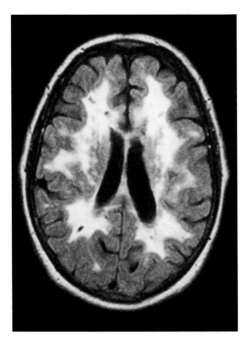

Figure 2.2 MRI scan of a 36-year-old woman with dementia, migraine and recurrent stroke-like episodes, as well as a family history of CADASIL. The scan shows extensive white matter changes and subcortical infarcts.

subcortical infarcts and leukoencephalopathy (CADASIL), an adult-onset hereditary disease affecting the tunica media of the small cerebral arteries, which has also been linked to the short arm of chromosome 19. Indeed, 25 missense mutations of the Notch3 gene on chromosome 19p13 have been identified in 90% of CADASIL patients. CADASIL is a rare but underdiagnosed illness with a progressive course and is characterized by migraine with aura and white matter hyperintensities on brain MRI (third to fourth decade), early stroke (fifth decade) and subcortical dementia due to diffuse leukoencephalopathy (sixth decade). Recent linkage to chromosome 19p13 in a family with typical autosomal-dominant migraine suggests the possible involvement of the Notch3 gene in some patients with otherwise typical migraine. Since 6% of migraine patients younger than 50 years with no vascular risk factors or autoimmune or demyelinating diseases have white matter hyperintensities on brain MRI, CADASIL should be suspected in patients with familial migraine, particularly when associated with prolonged aphasic and motor aura. Molecular diagnosis should be performed in all patients with autosomal-dominant migraine, prolonged atypical aura and white matter hyperintensities.

Epidemiology – Key points

- The International Headache Society has developed diagnostic criteria for migraine and tension headache.
- Using these criteria, migraine has been shown to affect 6% of males and 15% of females in the population, and tension headache 63% of males and 86% of females.
- There is a definite genetic component; it is believed to be multifactorial, but a locus on chromosome 19 relating to a calcium channel seems particularly important.

Key references

Breslau N, Davis GC, Andreski P. Migraine, psychiatric disorders, and suicide attempts: an epidemiologic study of young adults. *Psychiatry Res* 1991;37:11–23.

Chabriat H, Vahedi K, Iba-Zizen MT et al. Clinical spectrum of CADASIL: a study of 7 families. *Lancet* 1995;346:934–9.

Ducros A, Denier C, Joutel A et al. The clinical spectrum of familial hemiplegic migraine associated with mutations in a neuronal calcium gene. *N Engl J Med* 2001;345:17–24.

Göbel H, Petersen-Braun M, Soyka D. The epidemiology of headache in Germany: a nationwide survey of a representative sample on the basis of the headache classification of the International Headache Society. *Cephalalgia* 1994;14:97–106.

Headache Classification Committee of the International Headache Society. Classification and diagnostic criteria for headache disorders, cranial neuralgias and facial pain. *Cephalalgia* 1988;8(suppl 7):1–96.

Henry P, Michel P, Brochet B et al. A nationwide survey of migraine in France: prevalence and clinical features in adults. *Cephalalgia* 1992;12:229–37.

Hu XH, Markson LE, Lipton RB et al. Burden of migraine in the United States: disability and economic costs. *Arch Intern Med* 1999;159:813–18.

Joutel A, Bousser MG, Biousse V et al. A gene for familial hemiplegic migraine maps to chromosome 19. *Nat Genet* 1993;5:40–5.

Lipton RB, Diamond S, Reed M. Migraine diagnosis and treatment: results from the American Migraine Study II. *Headache* 2001;41:646–57.

O'Brien B, Goeree R, Streiner D. Prevalence of migraine headache in Canada: a population-based survey. *Int J Epidemiol* 1994;23:1020–6.

Ophoff RA, Terwindt GM, Vergouwe MN et al. Familial hemiplegic migraine and episodic ataxia type-2 are caused by mutations in the Ca^{2+} channel gene CACNL1A4. *Cell* 1996;87:543–52.

Osterhaus JT, Gutterman DL, Plachetka JR. Healthcare resource and lost labour costs of migraine headache in the US. *PharmacoEconomics* 1992;2:67–76.

Rasmussen BK, Jensen R, Schroll M et al. Epidemiology of headache in a general population – a prevalence study. *J Clin Epidemiol* 1991;44:1147–57.

Russell MB, Olesen J. Increased familial risk and evidence of genetic factor in migraine. *BMJ* 1995;311:541–4.

Stewart WF, Lipton RB, Celentano DD et al. Prevalence of migraine headache in the United States. Relation to age, income, race, and other sociodemographic factors. *JAMA* 1992;267:64–9.

Stewart WF, Lipton RB, Simon D. Work-related disability: results from the American migraine study. *Cephalalgia* 1996;16:231–8.

Terwindt GM, Ophoff RA, Haan J et al. Familial hemiplegic migraine; a clinical comparison of families linked and unlinked to chromosome 19. *Cephalalgia* 1996;16:153–5.

Vahlquist B. Migraine in children. *Int Arch Allergy* 1955;7:348–55.

Waters WE. The epidemiological enigma of migraine. *Int J Epidemiol* 1973;2:189–94.

Despite its pervasiveness and potential for significant disability, migraine has historically been under-recognized and under-treated. In the American Migraine Study conducted in 1989, only 16% of migraine sufferers identified by questionnaire had consulted a physician for headache in the previous year, and only 38% reported having ever been diagnosed with migraine by a physician. Although 96% of migraineurs used medications for their headaches, most (59%) used only over-the-counter rather than prescription medicines. The results of the American Migraine Study II demonstrate that although diagnosis of migraine has increased over the past decade, approximately half of migraineurs in the USA remain undiagnosed. Furthermore, the increases in consultation for and diagnosis of migraine have not been accompanied by increased use of prescription medicines for migraine management. Migraine continues to cause significant debilitation in sufferers, whether or not they are diagnosed by a physician, underscoring the need for healthcare professionals to recognize and effectively manage this important health problem.

Although the IHS criteria have proved invaluable for clinical research, the lack of their widespread implementation in clinical practice, or the strict implementation of the criteria, may contribute to the under-recognition of migraine. Migraine diagnosis does not consist simply in ruling out a secondary organic process but is effectively accomplished by understanding the clinical features and pattern of migraine. It is important to recognize that not one single criterion for migraine is necessary or sufficient for the diagnosis (Table 3.1). In other words, a patient with a bilateral non-throbbing headache may still have migraine if the headaches are moderately severe, associated with nausea, and worsened by routine physical activity. Headache specialists also recognize several non-IHS clinical features which are highly suggestive of migraine and aid in the recognition of the disorder

TABLE 3.1

Frequency of IHS migraine criteria

No single criterion necessary or sufficient for diagnosis of migraine

Characteristics (2/4)

- Unilateral 60%
- Throbbing 50%
- Moderate–severe intensity ~80%
- Pain worsened by routine physical activity > 95%

Associated symptoms (1/2)

- Nausea 86–95%, or vomiting 47–62%
- Photophobia 82–95%, phonophobia 61–98%

TABLE 3.2

Features of migraine not used by the IHS

- Predictable timing of headache around menstruation
- Stereotyped premonitory symptoms (mood changes, lethargy, photophobia, food cravings)
- Characteristic triggers (red wine, chocolate, stress, sleep or food deprivation)
- Positive family history of migraine
- Abatement with sleep
- Interferes with daily activities or ability to function
- Impaired ability to concentrate and difficulty with information processing
- Childhood migraine variants (cyclic abdominal pain, recurrent vertigo)

(Table 3.2). The diagnosis is therefore based on pattern recognition of a constellation of clinical features.

Tension-type headache is more common in the general population, but not necessarily in individuals seeking medical evaluation. Tension-type headaches are 'featureless' headaches which are classified mainly by the absence of migraine-associated features (Table 2.2). Patients are unlikely to seek medical attention for episodic tension-type headache or other mild non-disabling headache conditions. Patients generally effectively manage these headaches with lifestyle modifications or non-prescription analgesics. Patients with clinically relevant migraine often experience several different clinical presentations of headache including migraine, migrainous (not meeting all IHS criteria for migraine) and tension-type headache. This entire spectrum of headache activity responds equally well to migraine-specific (e.g. triptan) medications, suggesting that these different clinical presentations of headaches in migraine patients have a similar underlying biology. Therefore, although individual patients may have both tension-type headache and episodic migraine, the academic headache community no longer supports the concepts or use of the terms 'mixed headache disorder', 'tension-vascular headaches', 'vascular headaches' or 'muscle-contraction headaches'. The clinical caveat is that a patient with a recurrent, severe and stereotyped pattern of headaches of greater than 6 months' duration has migraine until proven otherwise.

Aura symptoms

Only a small proportion of patients have headaches preceded by auras, and their auras are not always consistent. It is also possible for aura symptoms to be experienced without significant headache. This may occur either during the evolution of more typical attacks over a patient's lifetime or occasionally de novo in older people when it may be difficult to differentiate migrainous auras from transient ischemic attacks.

Visual disturbances are the most common aura symptoms (Figure 3.1). Many migraine patients, even those without other symptoms, complain of photophobia and blurred vision, but the most characteristic aura symptoms are positive scintillations and visual loss. Scintillations are often formless 'flashing lights', but many patients describe a zig-zag disturbance expanding from the fixation point towards the periphery of vision, usually on one side over some 20 minutes, often leaving a scotoma inside it. Others experience one or more scotomata which may or may not overlie the fixation point, and total hemianopias are not

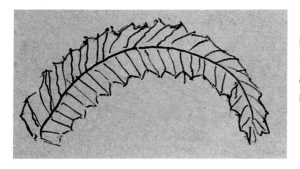

Figure 3.1
Migrainous visual disturbance drawn by a patient.

uncommon. The mechanism of the migrating scintillating scotoma is discussed in Chapter 4.

Sensory and other disturbances. Some people experience sensory disturbances, usually consisting of paresthesias rather than numbness, most commonly affecting the fingers and lips. Presumably such parts of the body are affected because they are represented by proportionally more of the cerebral cortex. Paresthesias in the legs are uncommon. The disturbance may move slowly from the fingers and the elbow over 10–20 minutes, far slower than that seen in focal epilepsy or a transient ischemic attack. Bilateral sensory disturbances often occur, occasionally compounded by hyperventilation. Motor weakness is less common than paresthesias. In most cases it follows the time course of the sensory disturbance, though some patients have a prolonged, familial type of hemiplegic migraine. Speech disturbances may be a feature of aura. Some people complain of a dysarthria, but most have dysphasias of presumed cortical origin, again usually lasting 20–30 minutes. They are often, but not always, associated with sensory disturbances in the dominant arm.

Location. The headache follows on the side opposite that of the aura symptoms in most patients, suggesting that intracerebral and extracerebral disturbances take place on the same side of the head. However, ipsilateral headache is surprisingly common, particularly in people referred to specialist clinics, presumably because they are considered to be unusual by the referring physician. Ipsilateral headache is even found in patients who collect information about their attacks on a prospective basis. Therefore, it is improbable that a direct connection exists between the aura symptoms and the headache site. It is more likely that both aura and headache reflect a common pathogenetic mechanism which produces each symptom on one or the other side of the head.

Complications of migraine

Death during a migraine attack is unusual, and there is some epidemiological evidence that the life expectancy of people with migraine is better than that of the general population. Stroke occurs occasionally, and many series of CT and MRI scans of patients with migraine and multiple auras show focal changes, suggesting infarction. There is, however, little correlation between this and the duration of attacks. Migraine appears to be a risk factor for stroke, particularly in conjunction with other risk factors, such as taking the contraceptive pill and smoking. In most cases, an alternative mechanism (for example, an arteriovenous malformation, atherosclerosis, hypercoagulable states, dissection of the carotid artery, or an embolism from the heart or great vessels) can be demonstrated, and is a more realistic explanation of the stroke than migraine alone. It is always prudent to scan a patient with fixed physical signs arising during a migraine attack, not only to establish the presence of a cerebral infarct but also because tumors and other lesions are occasionally found.

Migraine in children

Migraine attacks begin before the age of 10 years in about 20% of patients. However, most patients, particularly girls, develop migraine in their early teens. Headache in children has as many causes as that in adults, and it is more likely to be of structural origin in the young. Fever, meningitis, head injury, hydrocephalus and space-occupying lesions in the posterior fossa should be considered as possible causes. Many young children have attacks of periodic abdominal pain with nausea and vomiting which gradually turn into typical migrainous headaches as they grow older. Most of these children have a family history of migraine. There is also an association between migraine and travel sickness in childhood.

The prognosis of migraine in childhood is good. In one large, 30-year longitudinal study undertaken in Sweden, headaches resolved completely in one-third of patients, resolved but recurred later in life (perhaps in conjunction with the contraceptive pill) in another third and were consistent throughout adolescence and into adulthood in the remaining third. The excellent prognosis of migraine in children has made formal trials of prophylactic medication difficult, but most pediatric neurologists use either pizotifen (not available in the USA at time of press), amitriptyline, cyproheptadine or propranolol to prevent attacks if prophylactic treatment is clinically justified.

Clinical features of migraine and tension headaches – Key points

- A high proportion of patients with migraine self-medicate, and many have never been diagnosed by a physician.
- Aura symptoms, most commonly visual, but also sensory, speech and occasionally motor, are only seen in a minority of migraine patients, but are usually diagnostic.
- Permanent complications of migraine are rare.

Key references

Airy H. On a distinct form of transient hemiopsia. *Phil Trans R Soc* 1870;160:247–64.

Bille B. Migraine in childhood and its prognosis. *Cephalalgia* 1981;1:71–5.

Peatfield RC, Gawel MJ, Clifford Rose F. Asymmetry of the aura and pain in migraine. *J Neurol Neurosurg Psychiatry* 1981;44:846–8.

Lipton RB, Stewart WF. Migraine in the United States: a review of epidemiology and health care use. *Neurology* 1993;43(suppl 3):S6–S10.

Russell MB, Olesen J. A nosographic analysis of the migraine aura in a general population. *Brain* 1996;119: 355–61.

The underlying mechanisms of the migrainous headache, aura and associated symptoms are becoming better understood, though no unifying hypothesis has yet emerged.

The migraine aura

The term 'aura' has been used for nearly two thousand years to denote the sensory hallucinations immediately preceding certain epileptic seizures. For over a century, the term has been used to signify analogous symptoms which inaugurate certain migraine attacks. The transient neurological symptoms of the migraine aura are among the most striking features of migraine and frequently motivate patients to seek consultation with a physician. The most common aura is the visual hallucination which may take a variety of forms such as a dance of brilliant stars, sparks or flashes of light, blind spots, and complex geometric patterns. A variety of other symptoms may occur during the aura, including a tingling sensation often in the face and upper extremity, speech impairment or weakness of one side of the body (hemiparesis). These symptoms usually precede the headache phase by 20–60 minutes, and reflect focal dysfunction of brain cortex. According to the traditional vascular theory, the symptoms of the migraine aura are caused by vasoconstriction with resulting cerebral ischemia, while the aftercoming headache is a result of reflex vasodilation of large, cranial vessels as a response to the presumed ischemia of the constrictor phase.

However, many of the clinical features of migraine cannot be explained by the mechanism of ischemia of cerebral tissue espoused by the vascular theory.

- Aura is experienced by only approximately 15% of patients. Moreover, even in these patients, aura only occurs during some attacks.
- The majority of migraine patients report a constellation of premonitory features which precede the actual headache by hours or days. These include a variety of symptoms such as fluid retention,

thirst, food cravings, elation, depression and drowsiness. It would be impossible to account for these vegetative and affective symptoms on the basis of cerebral ischemia.

- Medications such as non-steroidal anti-inflammatory agents, neuroleptic agents and the anti-epileptic drug divalproex sodium, which have no vasoconstrictor activity, are extraordinarily effective in relieving the headache and associated symptoms during a migraine attack.

- The results from a variety of functional neuroimaging studies have shown only a small, albeit significant, decrease in cerebral blood flow (CBF) at the time of the migraine aura, in an area corresponding to the symptoms (Figure 4.1), which migrates across the cerebral cortex. The headache phase of migraine begins while CBF is still reduced, and the earliest phase of the aura is associated with an increase rather than a decrease in CBF.

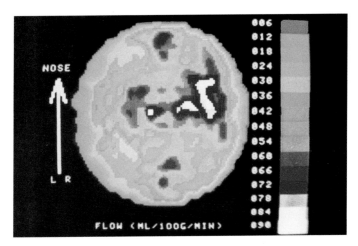

Figure 4.1 Cerebral blood flow tomogram of a patient with classical migraine. A 24-year-old woman with familial hemiplegic migraine arrived at the clinic with right scintillations, hemiparesis and aphasia. At the time of the study she had right arm paresthesias, left-sided headache, nausea and photophobia. The tomogram 5 cm above the orbitomeatal line shows reduced blood flow corresponding to the tomographic representation of left lateral temporal, parietal and frontal cortex. Reproduced with permission from Lauritzen M and Olesen J. *Brain* 1984;107:447.

The physician Lashley calculated that the growth of his own visual aura corresponded to an event moving across the cortex at a rate of 2–3 mm per minute. Earlier research by Leao had found that noxious stimulation of the exposed cerebral cortex of a rabbit produced a spreading decrease in electrical activity ('the spreading depression of Leao') that also moved across the cerebral cortex at a rate of 2–3 mm per minute. Some recent cerebral blood flow studies also suggest a wave moving at this speed. That the rates of spreading oligemia (reduction in CBF), visual aura and spreading cortical depression are equivalent strongly suggests that these phenomena may be related.

Curiously, this phase of spreading oligemia was preceded by a phase of focal hyperemia (increase in CBF) and did not respect the territory of single blood vessels. Therefore, it became highly unlikely that the reduction in CBF could be a result of vasoconstriction. It also became equally unlikely that the subsequent headache was a result of vasodilation, since the headache began during the time when CBF was still reduced. Similar changes in blood flow have been recently demonstrated using more sophisticated imaging modalities including positron emission tomography and high-field functional MRI, suggesting that cortical spreading depression (CSD) within human occipital cortex very likely explains the spatial and temporal characteristics of the migraine visual aura. The migraine aura seems not to be evoked by cerebral ischemia or vasoconstriction. It is more likely to be evoked by aberrant firing of neurons and related cellular changes characteristic of CSD, while blood-flow changes develop in response to fluctuations in neuronal activity during the visual aura.

The pathophysiological mechanism whereby spreading cortical depression is activated is unclear. However, there is a growing body of evidence to support the concept of central neuronal hyperexcitability, and thus a lowered threshold for activation, involving specialized neurons of the visual cortex. Evidence for central neuronal hyperexcitability comes from both neurophysiological and genetic studies. Transcranial magnetic studies of the occipital cortex in patients with migraine with aura have demonstrated that stimulation thresholds for the generation of phosphenes (visual 'sparks') are significantly reduced in migraine sufferers relative to control subjects with no history of migraine.

Genetic evidence supporting the concept of altered neuronal excitability has focused on abnormalities in neuronal calcium channels (Chapter 2), both in familial hemiplegic and typical migraine. It is postulated that alteration of the function of this channel may facilitate the initiation of aura through changes in the permeability of neurons to calcium, which results in an alteration of membrane polarity and a susceptibility to spontaneous or evoked depolarization and, thus, spreading cortical depression.

The migraine headache

Although our understanding of the underlying biology of migraine aura has been enormously enhanced by elegant functional neuroimaging studies during actual attacks, how this cortical event gives rise to headache is unclear. Furthermore, because aura occurs in only approximately 15–20% of patients, and only during some attacks even in these individuals, the genesis of the headache phase of migraine remains uncertain. It is, however, an area of ongoing and active investigation.

The central concepts in our current understanding of the pathogenesis of the head pain which occurs during a migraine attack are based on the anatomy and physiology of the trigeminovascular system. The pain during migraine is likely to result both from activation of the trigeminal nerve fibers which innervate pain-producing intracranial structures (large cerebral and dural blood vessels and the dura mater) as well as from a reduction in the function of the endogenous pain-control pathways that normally inhibit the transmission of pain to higher centers in the nervous system.

The trigeminal fibers that innervate the cerebral blood vessels arise from neurons within the trigeminal ganglion which contain substance P and calcitonin-gene-related peptide (CGRP). These neuropeptides are released when the trigeminal ganglion is stimulated in animals and humans, and jugular venous levels of CGRP are dramatically elevated in humans during acute attacks of migraine and cluster headache. It is generally accepted that the release of CGRP from trigeminal nerve endings leads to painful dilation of cerebral blood vessels. This leads to sensitization (activation) of these nerve fibers and subsequent

43

activation of central pain-transmitting and receiving neurons to which they connect. Ultimately, these signals are processed in the sensory cortex of the brain and perceived as the throbbing pain which has come to be regarded as one of the signature features of migraine.

Normally, ascending transmission of pain to the brain is modulated by a descending inhibitory pain-control system whose main constituents reside in the brainstem. In one of the most important and provocative studies in recent years in the field of migraine research, activation of the rostral (superior) brainstem was seen using positron emission tomography (PET) during migraine attacks without aura. Similarly, and unsurprisingly, other areas of the brain which are responsible for the normal processing of pain, including the cingulate, visual and auditory association cortices, were activated. The interesting finding was that the brainstem structures, but not the cortical structures, remained activated after resolution of the headache. This finding has been corroborated by a very recent study, and the area of activation corresponds to the same region confirmed to cause migraine-like headaches when stimulated in patients who had electrodes implanted for pain control for other conditions. These findings suggest that there are brainstem regions that play a pivotal role in either initiation or termination of the acute attack of migraine.

The regions which have been directly implicated as a result of these PET studies – the locus ceruleus, dorsal raphé and periaqueductal gray – are integral components in the endogenous pain-control network in humans. In addition, their activity may significantly affect blood flow to, and the metabolic function of, the occipital cortex. In experimental animals, stimulation of the locus ceruleus reduces CBF to the occipital cortex by 25%. Furthermore, the majority of ascending projections from the dorsal raphé nucleus terminate on neurons located within lamina 4 of the occipital cortex. In light of the preceding discussion of occipital cortical hyperexcitability, spreading cortical depression, and a spreading reduction in CBF which begins in the occipital cortex, it appears entirely plausible that these brainstem nuclei play a pivotal, if not defining, role in migraine.

Nitric oxide. Nitric oxide (NO), originating from the vascular endothelium, neurons and inflammatory cells (macrophages), is an important endogenous mediator of physiological vasodilation. Glyceryl trinitrate, which has been used for many years as a peripheral vasodilator in the treatment of angina pectoris, acts as an NO donor in vivo, and a transient headache is a common side-effect of its use. Olesen et al. demonstrated that patients with migraine, but not control subjects, developed a delayed headache resembling migraine 5–6 hours after the infusion of glyceryl trinitrate (Figure 4.2), suggesting that this pathway may also be an important mediator of migrainous headaches. Recently, CSD in animal models has been shown to cause upregulation of nitric oxide synthase (NOS), delayed (4–6 hours) inflammation of the dura and vasodilation. This provides the first plausible link between aura, neurogenic inflammation, and trigeminovascular activation – and, thus, headache. The delayed inflammatory reaction was inhibited by Type II NOS inhibitors, and it therefore provides a target for future drug development.

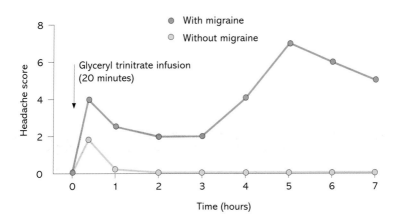

Figure 4.2 Comparison of mean headache scores in response to glyceryl trinitrate infusions (0.5 µg/kg/minute for 20 minutes) in people with and without migraine. Patients with migraine have a larger initial response to glyceryl trinitrate and a more marked delayed response than individuals without the condition. Reproduced with permission from Olesen J et al. 1994.

Mechanisms of migraine – Key points

* Migrainous aura symptoms are probably due to a wave of spreading depression moving across the appropriate part of the cerebral cortex; blood flow changes are secondary to this.
* The factors initiating the spreading depression, and its relationship to the mechanism of the headache, are poorly understood.
* PET scanning has shown an area in the brainstem that may initiate the migraine attack.

Key references

Bahra A, Matharu MS, Buchel C et al. Brainstem activation specific to migraine headache. *Lancet* 2001;357:1016–17.

Bolay H, Reuter, U, Dunn AK et al. Intrinsic brain activity triggers trigeminal meningeal afferents in a migraine model. *Nature Med* 2002;8:136–42.

Goadsby PJ, Edvinsson L, Ekman R. Vasoactive peptide release in the extracerebral circulation of humans during migraine headache. *Ann Neurol* 1990;28:183–7.

Igarashi H, Sakai F, Kan S et al. Magnetic resonance imaging of the brain in patients with migraine. *Cephalalgia* 1991;11:69–74.

Kaube H, Hoskin KL, Goadsby PJ. Activation of the trigeminovascular system by mechanical distension of the superior sagittal sinus in the cat. *Cephalalgia* 1992;12:133–6.

Lauritzen M. Pathophysiology of the migraine aura. The spreading depression theory. *Brain* 1994;117:199–210.

MacLennan SJ, Martin GR. Actions of non-peptide ergot alkaloids at 5-HT_1-like and 5-HT_2 receptors mediating vascular smooth muscle contraction. *Arch Pharmacol* 1990; 342:120–9.

Moskowitz MA. Neurogenic inflammation in the pathophysiology and treatment of migraine. *Neurology* 1993;43(suppl 3):S16–20.

Olesen J, Friberg L, Olsen TS et al. Timing and topography of cerebral blood flow, aura, and headache during migraine attacks. *Ann Neurol* 1990;28:791–8.

Olesen J, Thomsen LL, Iversen H. Nitric oxide is a key molecule in migraine and other vascular headaches. *Trends Pharmacol Sci* 1994;15:149–53.

Reuter U, Chiarugi A, Bolay H, Moskowitz MA. Nuclear factor-κB as a molecular target for migraine therapy. *Ann Neurol* 2002;51: 507–16.

Weiller C, May A, Limmroth V et al. Brain stem activation in spontaneous human migraine attacks. *Nature Med* 1995;1:658–60.

Most attacks of migraine are assumed to arise spontaneously through an intrinsic brainstem mechanism sometimes triggered by external factors. Many patients report that their headaches are triggered by stress or, more commonly, by the cessation of stress, such as at a weekend or on the first day of a holiday. The pathophysiological basis for the influence of stress on migraine is unclear, but there is evidence that the most important brain circuit which contributes to analgesia in humans, which includes the amygdala, periaqueductal gray, dorsolateral pontine tegmentum and the rostroventromedial medulla in the brainstem, may be modulated by acute stress or the expectation of relief. Through descending projections, this circuit controls both spinal and trigeminal dorsal horn pain transmission neurons and mediates both opioid- and stimulation-produced analgesia. Several different neurotransmitters are involved in the modulatory actions of this circuit, which could provide a physiological mechanism for the pain-modulating actions of mood, attention and expectation.

Female hormones

The importance of female hormones as triggering factors in migrainous attacks is evident from the sharp rise in headache prevalence seen at puberty in women but not in men, and by the influence of the female hormonal cycles on the frequency and severity of headaches.

Female menstrual cycle. Many adult women say that their headaches predictably occur and are worse before or at the time of menstruation. Some women have attacks only at this time, and a few even need to be told that headache is not an invariable feature of a menstrual period. A recent study in Italy compared the clinical features and response to treatment of menstrual and non-menstrual attacks of migraine in women with menstrually related migraine. They demonstrated that migraine attacks occurring on the first 2 days of the cycle are longer, more severe and less responsive to analgesics than non-menstrual attacks in women with menstrually related migraine. There is considerable evidence that headache attacks are triggered by falling estrogen levels. High-dose supplementation with exogenous estrogen towards the end of the menstrual cycle postpones both the period and the associated headache (Figure 5.1). Some patients are helped by receiving a small dose of estrogen a day or two before menstruation. This gives a 'soft landing' to the estrogen level, while permitting the menstrual period to take place.

With few exceptions, migrainous attacks tend to improve during pregnancy, particularly after the first trimester, as hormone levels become stable. However, attacks are common about 1 week postpartum, the time of a precipitous drop in estrogen levels.

The contraceptive pill. Some women find their migraine is worsened by the contraceptive pill. This applies particularly to combined estrogen/progesterone preparations in which an artificially high estrogen level is

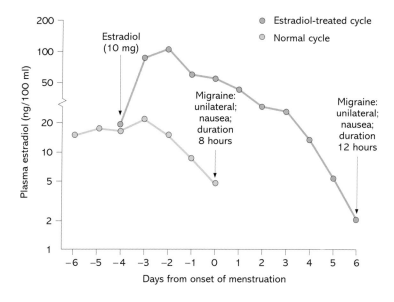

Figure 5.1 The effect of estradiol in postponing both periods and headache is the best evidence linking menstrual attacks to falling estrogen levels. Reproduced, with permission, from Somerville BW 1972.

maintained for 3 weeks each month. When the pills are stopped, hormones fall rapidly to low levels in order to trigger a withdrawal bleed. This association applies to all migrainous headaches whether or not they are preceded by an aura.

Considerable epidemiological evidence supports an association between the combined oral contraceptive pill and stroke in women with migraine preceded by an aura, particularly if they also smoke. Most authorities feel that the combined contraceptive pill is contraindicated under these circumstances.

No systematic studies have been undertaken examining the effects of the progesterone-only contraceptive pill on migraine. These preparations carry no thrombotic risk, so their absolute contraindication in the presence of a migrainous aura cannot be applied.

Hormone replacement therapy (HRT). Migraine headaches may become worse at the time of the menopause. Percutaneous HRT preparations contain about as much estrogen as that found in the contraceptive pill and may worsen, rather than improve, migraine. Oral conjugated estrogen preparations may affect migraine less than other non-conjugated forms, yet still suppress distressing hot flushes and other estrogen deficiency symptoms. Some women, however, tolerate synthetic percutaneous estrogen better. Patients should receive preparations containing the lowest dose of estrogen able to suppress these menopausal symptoms, and it is unrealistic to expect any form of HRT to have a beneficial effect on migraine.

Hormonal treatment. With the exception of the relationship between migrainous auras and the combined contraceptive pill, decisions regarding hormonal treatment in people with migraine should be made by the patients themselves after discussion of all available information. Many authorities, however, argue that patients presenting to neurologists because of frequent, distressing migraine attacks should be advised to discontinue taking the contraceptive pill rather than undergo prophylactic drug therapy to suppress their headaches. There is certainly a place for short-term drug treatment, as the adverse effects of the pill often take several months to cease after it is discontinued.

Food and drink

About 20% of patients attending the Princess Margaret Migraine Clinic (London, UK) report that migrainous headaches are triggered by foods, such as cheese, chocolate and citrus fruits. Most are sensitive to all three foods and few to only one. Associations of migraine with other foods are tenuous. Few patients have headaches only when triggered by these three foods, but most have spontaneous attacks even when they assiduously avoid all the triggering factors identified.

Most information on the link between migraine and foods has been assembled from epidemiological surveys. The results of a few small challenge studies have been published confirming these observations, though these have only been carried out on highly selected patients. Many people are also sensitive to alcoholic drinks – some to alcohol in general and others to specific beverages, such as red wine, fortified wines or beer. There is an imperfect correlation between sensitivity to red wine and food, but many patients feel they are affected by only one of these. There is no justification for a patient to eliminate food from their diet that has not been specifically identified as a migraine precipitant.

It is unlikely that closely correlated responses to such disparate foodstuffs are immunologically mediated. Extensive studies of circulating antibodies in diet-sensitive patients with migraine failed to confirm abnormalities of IgE or IgG. In addition, no significantly different, consistent responses have been seen in skin tests compared with those from the general population. Many of the foods implicated have been fermented, and attention has been devoted to small molecules found in such foods. The first agent suggested was tyramine, which produced headache in sensitive subjects in challenge studies undertaken by Hanington some years ago. However, tyramine is not found in all implicated foods, and other transmitters, including flavonoid polyphenols (contributing, for example, to the pigment in wine), may also be important. Although significant deficiencies in enzymatic pathways for the detoxification of these substances have been found in diet-sensitive people with migraine, attention is currently focused on the direct pharmacological effects of these substances on serotonergic and other systems. It will be clear that, as yet, these mechanisms remain poorly understood.

The induction of headache by large quantities of alcohol (hangover) is discussed in Chapter 1. Most patients seeking advice about spontaneous migraine attacks and who report sensitivity to, for example, red wine say that a single glass will trigger a headache identical to spontaneous ones.

Precipitating causes – Key points

- Migraine attacks often seem to be related to relaxation after stress.
- Falling estrogen levels, either in normal cycles or due to contraceptive pills or HRT, can also trigger migraine.
- About a fifth of sufferers report that attacks can be precipitated by cheese, chocolate, or alcoholic drinks – the mechanism of this is probably chemical but is as yet poorly understood.

Key references

Bousser M-G. Migraine, female hormones and stroke. *Cephalalgia* 1999;19:75–9.

De Lignières B, Vincens M, Mauvais-Jarvis P et al. Prevention of menstrual migraine by percutaneous estradiol. *BMJ* 1986;293:1540.

Granella F et al. 2001 Characteristics of menstrual and non-menstrual attacks in women with menstrually related migraine. *Cephalalgia* 2001;21:263–4.

Peatfield RC, Hussain N, Glover VAS et al. Prostacyclin, tyramine, and red wine. In: Olesen J, Moskowitz MA, eds. *Experimental Headache Models.* Philadelphia: Lippincott-Raven, 1995:267–76.

Somerville BW. The role of estradiol withdrawal in the etiology of menstrual migraine. *Neurology* 1972;22:355–65.

Tzourio C, Tehindrazanarivelo A, Iglésias S et al. Case-control study of migraine and risk of ischaemic stroke in young women. *BMJ* 1995;310:830–3.

Most drug therapies discussed in this chapter are effective, to various extents, against the headache and associated symptoms of a migraine attack. Drugs are also available to suppress nausea and vomiting. However, no drug therapies are specifically aimed at aura symptoms, though these are seldom the most prominent cause of a patient's distress. It has been reported that rebreathing (for example, into a paper bag) can shorten the aura phase of a migrainous attack.

Many people never seek medical advice about headaches, and presumably simple analgesics, such as aspirin, paracetamol, ibuprofen or low-dose compound codeine preparations, provide satisfactory relief. Nevertheless, recent epidemiological surveys in the USA reveal that many individuals not seeking medical advice about their headaches fulfill the IHS definition of migraine, and that the same number again have 'severe, non-migrainous headache' (Figure 6.1). Significant numbers of patients, therefore, do not seek advice about disabling attacks.

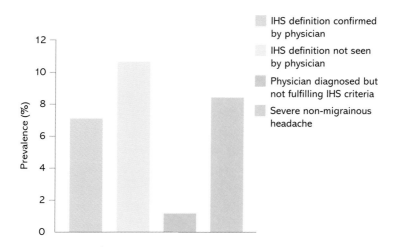

IHS definition confirmed by physician

IHS definition not seen by physician

Physician diagnosed but not fulfilling IHS criteria

Severe non-migrainous headache

Figure 6.1 Prevalence of migraine over 1 year in about 10 750 females aged 12–80 years. Adapted with permission from Lipton RB et al. 1992.

General principles

The objectives of acute migraine therapy are to restore the patient to normal function by rapidly and consistently alleviating pain and the associated symptoms of nausea and vomiting, without recurrence of pain within 24 hours, and with minimal or no adverse events. Abortive migraine medications can be either migraine specific or non-specific (Table 6.1); the former are only effective in alleviating headache and not other pain disorders. The choice of medication and route of administration depends on the severity and frequency of headache, the timing and intensity of associated symptoms, and the patient's prior experience with over-the-counter non-specific agents, as almost all patients will have tried one or more of these prior to seeking medical advice.

Because migraine severity varies considerably between individuals as well as within the same individual from attack to attack, a 'cookbook' or step care approach to acute therapy is inappropriate. In step care, treatment is escalated after first-line medications fail. In stratified care, initial treatment is based on measurement of the severity of illness, as with most other disease states in medicine. Stratified care is based on the principle that patient characteristics (e.g. headache-related disability as measured by the MIDAS disability rating instrument) can be used to determine an individual patient's treatment needs, thereby increasing the chance of successful therapy from the outset. Results from the first controlled trial which evaluated these strategies of care for the acute treatment of migraine indicate that stratified care provides significantly better clinical outcomes than step care strategies within or across attacks, as measured by headache response and disability time.

Non-steroidal anti-inflammatory drugs

The majority of migraine sufferers self-treat their headaches with non-prescription analgesics. Recently, a number of non-prescription NSAIDs have been approved for treatment of mild-to-moderate migraine, and these remain the mainstay of clinical management, at least in general or family practice. The best trials have been conducted with aspirin, ibuprofen, diclofenac or naproxen sodium, and smaller ones with tolfenamic acid. Patients usually respond better to a soluble drug preparation than to a sustained-release formulation designed for the suppression of chronic arthritic pain. Patients should be advised not to take these drugs on an empty stomach, to reduce the risk of dyspepsia. Indomethacin is less effective in the management of migraine than other NSAIDs, and sometimes induces headache as a side-effect of chronic medication. It does, however, have a role in the management of chronic paroxysmal hemicrania (see Chapter 9).

Opioid analgesics

Most neurologists avoid the use of potentially addictive analgesics, for example morphine and pethidine (meperidine), for a benign recurrent condition such as migraine. Nevertheless drugs such as codeine, dihydrocodeine and dextropropoxyphene are taken extensively for a wide variety of pain syndromes, often in compound preparations with aspirin or paracetamol and sometimes with an antiemetic as well. Whereas these drugs are highly effective for short-term use, their daily administration, particularly if combined with caffeine, can cause a consistent, daily headache. These drugs, therefore, are not encouraged as first-line interventions except for patient populations who are poor candidates for $5\text{-}HT_1$-agonist therapy (such as the pregnant or those with high cardiovascular risk).

Patients taking these preparations often improve dramatically if told to discontinue their analgesic completely, though no properly controlled studies of this phenomenon have been carried out. It is unlikely that patients taking pure aspirin or paracetamol can induce a drug-abuse headache, and there is evidence that NSAIDs taken continuously have prophylactic properties in patients with migraine.

Antiemetics

The nausea and vomiting often seen in severe migrainous attacks are reflected in gastric stasis, which inhibits the absorption of medication taken by mouth. This may be true even if no vomiting takes place. Antiemetics, such as metoclopramide and domperidone, have a modest effect in increasing the absorption of oral medications as well as relieving nausea, whereas phenothiazine antiemetics tend to delay analgesic absorption. Many compound preparations containing simple analgesics and metoclopramide are now available, and these should be used in preference to phenothiazines unless sedation is also intended.

Ergotamine

Ergotamine, an active ingredient of the ergot fungus that grows on rye, has been a mainstay in the management of severe migrainous headache for around 100 years. It has a complex pharmacology, involving interaction with a wide variety of serotonin receptors, as well as alpha adrenergic receptors and others. It is very poorly absorbed (less than 3%) by mouth, but this is improved if it is given as a suppository or inhaled. The preparation for parenteral injection was unstable, and the inhaled preparation contained CFC propellants, so both have now been withdrawn in many countries. Ergotamine is believed to have a vasoconstrictor effect on inflamed dilated blood vessels, but it also penetrates the blood–brain barrier and affects trigeminal relay pathways in the brainstem.

Most of the clinical trials using ergotamine in migraine were undertaken many years ago on small numbers of patients, and the results are inconclusive by modern statistical standards. Ergotamine's former role has largely been taken over by sumatriptan, but it still has a place in the management of prolonged, infrequent, disabling migraine attacks.

In gross overdose, ergotamine produces peripheral vasoconstriction and gangrene. It has recently become clear that patients can become dependent on as little as 0.5 mg daily of ergotamine, developing a severe rebound headache after each dose, and they gain only short-term relief by repeating treatment. If these patients stop using ergotamine completely they develop a very severe headache lasting for about a week, but are much better thereafter.

Dihydroergotamine, also a potent vasoconstrictor, is barely absorbed orally, but is available for parenteral and nasal administration. A lower incidence of nausea and vomiting, and probably of rebound headache, is associated with its use. A recent trial of the nasal preparation has shown its effectiveness to be comparable to that of sumatriptan and substantially greater than that of placebo. Dihydroergotamine has been popular in the USA and some countries in Europe.

The sympathomimetic amine isometheptene has a vasoconstrictor action and has a modest clinical effect in migraine attacks.

Selective 5-HT$_1$ agonists (triptans)

Triptans are selective 5-HT$_{1B}$ and 5-HT$_{1D}$ receptor agonists, and some are agonists at the 5-HT$_{1F}$ receptor. These drugs are believed to constrict extracerebral intracranial vessels (via 5-HT$_{1B}$ receptors), inhibit activity in peripheral trigeminal neurons (5-HT$_{1D/1F}$), and block transmission in the trigeminal nucleus (5-HT$_{1D/1F}$). The US Headache Consortium Guidelines and recent triptan meta-analyses have concluded that all of the triptans are effective and are indicated for patients whose migraine attacks are associated with moderate to significant disability or who fail to respond to other medications. Triptans relieve head pain and also the associated symptoms of nausea, vomiting, photophobia and phonophobia. They are most effective when administered while the pain is mild.

Available triptans. Sumatriptan was the first triptan to be developed, followed by zolmitriptan, naratriptan, rizatriptan, almotriptan, frovatriptan and eletriptan.

Sumatriptan is available in an injectable preparation (6 mg subcutaneously), a nasal spray (20 mg), tablets (25, 50 or 100 mg) and, in a few countries, a suppository (25 mg). Subcutaneous sumatriptan has a very rapid onset of action, reaching peak plasma concentrations within 12 minutes. Peak plasma concentrations of oral sumatriptan are reached in 2 hours. Sumatriptan is metabolized principally by monoamine oxidase (MAO) A, and its use as an oral or nasal spray formulation is therefore contraindicated in patients taking MAO inhibitors. Placebo-controlled trials have consistently shown that subcutaneous sumatriptan (6 mg), oral sumatriptan and sumatriptan nasal spray are effective. Subcutaneous sumatriptan, 6 mg, had on average a 69% response at 1 hour. Intranasal sumatriptan, 20 mg, had on average a 61% response at 2 hours. A recent triptan meta-analysis by Ferrari et al. uses oral sumatriptan, 100 mg, as the standard, with a 2-hour headache response of 59% (95% CI: 57–61).

Zolmitriptan is more lipophilic than sumatriptan. It is available as 2.5 and 5 mg tablets, as 2.5 and 5 mg orally disintegrating tablets, and as a 5 mg nasal spray. The meta-analysis demonstrated a headache response at 2 hours of 64% for the 2.5 mg dose and 66% for the 5 mg dose. Zolmitriptan nasal spray, 5 mg, provides rapid onset of relief of migraine, with the first signs of efficacy apparent within 15 minutes. Response rates on headache for 5 mg zolmitriptan nasal spray are significantly higher than for the oral tablet formulation, 2.5 mg, from 15 minutes up to and including 2 hours. Headache response at 2 hours was 70% for the 5 mg zolmitriptan nasal spray.

Naratriptan is available as 1 mg (in the USA and some other countries) and 2.5 mg tablets. The recommended dose is 2.5 mg. Naratriptan is excreted largely as unchanged drug in the urine. The meta-analysis demonstrated a headache response at 2 hours of 49%. The side-effect profile of naratriptan is generally equal to that of placebo in controlled trials, and recurrence rate on average was 21.4%, which is among the lowest within this class of medications.

Rizatriptan is available as an oral tablet and as a rapidly dissolving wafer (5 mg, 10 mg). The recommended oral dose is 10 mg, except in patients who are taking propranolol, for whom the recommended dose is 5 mg. Rizatriptan is metabolized principally by MAOA, with metabolites being excreted in the urine. Coadministration with propranolol results in an increase in the plasma concentration of rizatriptan. It should not be used by patients taking MAO inhibitors. The meta-analysis demonstrated headache response at 2 hours of 62% and 69% for the 5 mg and 10 mg dose, respectively. Rizatriptan also appears from randomized controlled trials to possess a high consistency of effect from attack to attack.

Almotriptan is available as a 12.5 mg tablet; it is also available as a 6.25 mg tablet in the USA and some other countries. The recommended initial dose is 12.5 mg, which can be repeated after 2 hours if the headache returns. No more than two doses should be used in a 24-hour period. It is partially metabolized in the liver (by MAO 27%, P450 [3A4 and 2D6] 12%) to inactive metabolites. Almotriptan has no significant interaction with propranolol, selective serotonin reuptake inhibitors, or MAO inhibitors. The meta-analysis demonstrated a headache response of 61% at 2 hours. Almotriptan, like naratriptan, has a tolerability profile comparable to that of placebo.

Frovatriptan is available as a 2.5 mg tablet in the USA and some other countries. A second dose may be taken for headache recurrence. The total daily dose should not exceed three tablets. It is metabolized in the liver (by P4540 [CYP 1A2]) and excreted in the urine. The mean half-life is 26 hours, which is 4–12 times that of any other triptan. The meta-analysis demonstrated a headache response at 2 hours of 42% with a very good side-effect profile – comparable to that of placebo.

Eletriptan is available as 40 mg and 80 mg tablets. Eletriptan is metabolized by CP3A4 and therefore has the potential for interactions with drugs metabolized by this enzyme system. Whether there are clinically relevant drug interactions is uncertain. The meta-analysis demonstrated headache response at 2 hours of 60% and 66% for the 40 mg and 80 mg dose, respectively. Adverse events appeared to be more common with eletriptan than with other triptans such as sumatriptan, naratriptan, almotriptan and frovatriptan.

Selection of drug and formulation. In summary, therefore, seven triptans – sumatriptan, zolmitriptan, naratriptan, rizatriptan, almotriptan, frovatriptan and eletriptan – in a variety of formulations are currently available. They are safe, effective and appropriate as first-line therapy for the patient who has a moderate to severe migraine headache or as second-line therapy for those for whom an adequate trial of NSAIDs or other non-opiate analgesics has failed to provide adequate relief in the past. No evidence supports their use during the aura phase of a migraine attack. All are relatively expensive, though costs vary between drugs and in different countries and can fluctuate considerably within countries.

When determining which triptan to use, it is important to keep in mind that the response to any triptan is idiosyncratic. Despite similar receptor targets, it is well known that individual patients may have a robust response to one triptan but only a partial or complete lack of response to another. With few exceptions, matching the pharmacokinetic attributes of a medication to the clinical characteristics of a typical attack is therefore an inexact science. Individual patient

> **Acute treatment – Key points**
>
> - Non-steroidal anti-inflammatory drugs and gastrokinetic antiemetics should usually be analgesics of first choice.
> - Short-term opiates (e.g. codeine) can be useful, but their chronic administration can lead to a dull background headache.
> - Triptans, agonists at $5\text{-}HT_{1B}$ and $5\text{-}HT_{1D}$ receptors, are highly effective as analgesics, though expensive.

preference is complex and depends on a balance of attributes that is unique to each patient. The formulation has been proven to be more important than the chemical entity. Subcutaneous sumatriptan is still the most effective agent, but its use is limited by patients' aversion to injections.

Several oral triptans can provide headache relief within 30–60 minutes (almotriptan, eletriptan, sumatriptan, rizatriptan, zolmitriptan) when patients require efficacy and speed of onset of acute migraine therapy. When the headache intensifies very quickly (< 30 minutes), or nausea and vomiting are early and severe associated symptoms, a non-oral route of administration is appropriate. Subcutaneous injection is fastest and most effective. The nasal spray formulation may provide a faster onset of action than the oral, but is often associated with a disagreeable taste. Zolmitriptan nasal spray provides fast relief, as early as 15 minutes, and appears to have a less disagreeable taste than sumatriptan nasal spray. Almotriptan, naratriptan or frovatriptan are appropriate choices for patients who are prone to triptan-related side-effects.

Ultimately, the triptan of choice is the one that restores the patient's ability to function, by swiftly and consistently relieving pain and associated symptoms with a minimum of side-effects and without recurrence of symptoms. If patients are made aware of these treatment expectations, finding the ideal triptan may ultimately depend upon the ability of an individual to try several different treatment options, each for more than one attack. Patients evaluate their individual treatment by weighing efficacy, onset of action, duration, reliability, tolerability, ease of use, and general sense of well-being. While clinical trials examine only efficacy at specified points in time within populations of patients, this type of individual preference trial may provide a more accurate assessment of which triptan is best for a particular individual.

Key references

Cutler N, Mushet GR, Davis R et al. Oral sumatriptan for the acute treatment of migraine: evaluation of three dosage strengths. *Neurology* 1995;45(suppl 7):S5–9.

Ferrari MD, Roon KI, Lipton RB, Goadsby PJ. Oral triptans (serotonin 5-HT$_{1B/1D}$ agonists) in acute migraine treatment: a meta-analysis of 53 trials. *Lancet* 2001;358: 1668–75.

Goadsby PJ. A triptan too far? *J Neurol Neurosurg Psychiatry* 1998;64:143–7.

Hakkarainen H, Vapaatalo H, Gothoni G et al. Tolfenamic acid is as effective as ergotamine during migraine attacks. *Lancet* 1979;2: 326–8.

Lipton RB, Stewart WF, Celentano DD et al. Undiagnosed migraine headaches. *Arch Intern Med* 1992; 152:1273–8.

Lipton RB, Stewart WF, Stone AM et al. Stratified care vs step care strategies for migraine. The Disability in Strategies of Care (DISC) study: a randomized trial. *JAMA* 2000; 284:2599–605.

Lipton RB, Stewart WF, Cady RK et al. 2000 Wolff Award. Sumatriptan for the range of headaches in migraine sufferers: results of the Spectrum Study. *Headache* 2000;40: 783–91.

Olesen J. Analgesic headache. *BMJ* 1995;310:479–80.

Pascual J et al. Consistent efficacy and tolerability of almotriptan in the acute treatment of multiple migraine attacks: results of a large, randomised, double-blind placebo controlled study. *Cephalalgia* 2000;20:588–96.

Plosker GL, McTavish D. Sumatriptan. A reappraisal of its pharmacology and therapeutic efficacy in the acute treatment of migraine and cluster headache. *Drugs* 1994;47:622–51.

Subcutaneous Sumatriptan International Study Group. Treatment of migraine attacks with sumatriptan. *N Engl J Med* 1991; 325:316–21.

Teall J, Tuchman M, Cutler N et al. Rizatriptan (Maxalt) for the acute treatment of migraine and migraine recurrence. A placebo controlled outpatient study. *Headache* 1998; 38:281–7.

Tfelt-Hansen P, Henry P, Mulder LJ et al. The effectiveness of combined oral lysine acetylsalicylate and metoclopramide compared with oral sumatriptan for migraine. *Lancet* 1995;346:923–6.

Tfelt-Hansen P et al. Ergotamine in the acute treatment of migraine; a review and European consensus. *Brain* 2000;123:9–18.

Tfelt-Hansen P, De Vries P, Saxena PR. Triptans in migraine: a comparative review of pharmacology, pharmacokinetics and efficacy. *Drugs* 2000;60:1259–87.

Touchon JA on behalf of the study group. A comparison of intranasal dihydroergotamine (DHE) and subcutaneous sumatriptan 6 mg in the acute treatment of migraine. In: Olesen J, Tfelt-Hansen P, eds. *Headache Treatment: Trial Methodology and New Drugs.* Philadelphia: Lippincott-Raven, 1997:213–18.

Welch KMA, Mathew NT, Stone P et al. Tolerability of sumatriptan: clinical trials and post-marketing experience. *Cephalalgia* 2000; 20(8):687–95.

Prophylactic treatment

Prophylaxis against migraine headaches has several objectives:

- to decrease the frequency, severity and duration of migraine attacks
- to make attacks more responsive to acute treatments
- to improve the quality of life of migraine sufferers.

Appropriate indications for prophylaxis are given in Table 7.1. Although it has been suggested that a specific number of migraine attacks should determine the threshold for initiating preventive therapy, a more reasonable approach may be to consider the degree of impairment patients experience with recurring migraines, regardless of their exact frequency. Patients with contraindications to acute treatment, those in whom acute therapy no longer provides relief, and patients who manifest side-effects to acute therapy are also candidates for preventive therapy. Patients themselves may prefer prophylaxis. Another important reason for instituting migraine prophylaxis is the presence of uncommon conditions such as familial hemiplegic migraine or migrainous cerebral infarction that might result in neurological damage. The presence of comorbid conditions in patients with migraine

TABLE 7.1

Indications for migraine prophylaxis

- Frequent headaches or recurring migraine that in the patient's opinion significantly interfere with activities despite acute treatment

- Contraindication to, or failure or overuse of, acute therapies

- Adverse events with acute therapies

- The cost of both acute and preventive therapies

- Patient preference

- Presence of uncommon migraine conditions, including hemiplegic migraine, basilar migraine, migraine with prolonged aura or migrainous infarction (to prevent neurological damage – as based on expert consensus) headache should also lower the threshold for instituting prophylaxis, including cardiovascular diseases such as hypertension or fibromyalgia, neurological comorbidities such as epilepsy, gastrointestinal conditions such as functional bowel disorders, psychiatric manifestations such as depression or mania, and other conditions such as asthma or allergies.

Patients who are candidates for migraine prophylaxis also require acute medication. Both are necessary for long-term management, and patients should be educated to understand the difference between these treatments and when to use each. Setting realistic expectations is very important in ensuring compliance with prophylactic therapy. At least 2 months of therapy at a therapeutic dosage is required to evaluate the effectiveness of any prophylactic medication, and patients must understand that control, not cure or complete suppression of attacks, is the primary goal. It is also important for patients to realize that, even with prophylaxis, acute attacks may and often do still occur, requiring the concomitant use of acute therapy. They should also understand that use of prophylactic medications to treat acute attacks is an ineffective approach to treatment and is not why these medications have been prescribed.

For migraine prophylaxis, physicians may choose from several classes of agents, taking into account their efficacy, dosing requirements, contraindications, drug interactions and side-effect profiles. Prophylactic agents for migraine include β-blockers, calcium channel blockers, tricyclic antidepressants, selective serotonin reuptake inhibitors (SSRIs), serotonin antagonists, non-steroidal anti-inflammatory drugs (NSAIDs), antiepileptic drugs and a variety of miscellaneous agents (Table 7.2).

Beta-blockers

Beta-blockers are efficacious for the prevention of migraine headache and may be particularly useful in migraineurs who also have hypertension or angina. These agents, however, should be avoided in those with asthma, congestive heart failure, insulin-dependent diabetes, Raynaud's disease or depression. Only propranolol and timolol are approved by the Food and Drug Administration (FDA) for the prevention of migraine headache, but nadalol, metoprolol and atenolol

TABLE 7.2

Conventional migraine prophylactic drugs

The medications are listed in the table in the approximate order in which they should be used in a typical patient

Drug	Daily adult dose (mg)	
	Start	Maximum
Propranolol	80	320
Atenolol	50	150
Pizotifen	0.5	3.0
Sodium valproate	400	1000
Methysergide	0.5	6.0
Naproxen	250	1000
Amitriptyline	10–25	100

have all been shown to be effective. Nadolol and atenolol are preferred by some because of their longer elimination half-lives, which allow for once-daily dosing. They may also have a somewhat more favorable side-effect profile than other more lipophilic β-blockers. Beta-blockers with intrinsic sympathomimetic activity are ineffective. The mechanism of action of these agents in preventing migraine headache is not well understood. Common side-effects seen with β-blockers include orthostatic hypotension, fatigue, depression and sexual dysfunction. It may be possible to manage side-effects while keeping patients on β-blocker therapy by adjusting dosages, switching to an alternate β-blocker or changing the time of therapy. Medications with the potential for drug interactions with β-blockers include rizatriptan and calcium channel blockers.

Serotonin antagonists

Pizotifen (which is not available in the USA), methysergide and cyproheptadine have been used successfully for migraine prophylaxis. Methysergide has perhaps the best reputation for abolishing migrainous attacks completely, even when it is given to patients previously unresponsive to both pizotifen and propranolol. Initially, doses of up to

65

12 mg/day were used. This produced retroperitoneal fibrosis and thickening of the cardiac valves in some patients. Usually, however, these fibrotic changes regress if the drug is stopped. More recent studies use a maximum of 6 mg/day for no more than 6 consecutive months before the drug is stopped for 1 month, and the risk of retroperitoneal fibrosis seems negligible. Many patients respond to doses smaller than this. One other significant side-effect, found in women in particular, is leg pain that is minimized by introducing the drug slowly, starting with 0.5 mg/day for a few days before building up towards the full dose. Serotonin antagonists, particularly pizotifen, also have sedating properties and may induce weight gain. Some authorities feel it is prudent to avoid the use of triptans, ergotamine and dihydroergotamine as acute migraine therapy in patients receiving serotonin antagonists, particularly methysergide since its active metabolite is also a 5-HT$_{1B/1D}$ agonist.

Calcium channel blockers

This class of agents may be the least effective in migraine prevention, though a small subset of patients using these drugs appear to do well. Verapamil has seen the most use in the USA, and the longer-acting agent flunarizine is commonly used in continental Europe. Candidates for prophylaxis with calcium channel blockers include patients with hypertension, angina or asthma, especially where β-blockers are relatively contraindicated. Calcium channel blockers are also used in patients with a history of prolonged aura, migrainous infarction or vestibular migraine with vertigo. They may be the best-tolerated of migraine prophylactic agents, with few side-effects (constipation is the most common); however, they are also probably the least efficacious. If patients treated with a calcium channel blocker do not improve after 2–3 months, it may be prudent to switch to another class of agents. The potential for drug interaction exists with β-blockers.

Tricyclic antidepressants

Tricyclic antidepressants are used for migraine prophylaxis, although only amitriptyline has been shown to be substantially more efficacious than placebo in controlled studies. Nortriptyline and doxepin are also used for migraine prophylaxis. Nortriptyline is the major metabolite of amitriptyline, and is generally associated with fewer CNS side-effects. A recent meta-analysis identified 38 placebo-controlled trials that have evaluated the efficacy of antidepressants for the treatment of migraine and tension-type headache. Patients receiving tricyclic antidepressants were twice as likely to report improvement, with about 1 patient in 3 treated reporting improvement. As for specific medications, at present only amitriptyline has been studied in sufficient numbers of patients to demonstrate statistically significant benefits. Tricyclic antidepressants are generally used in lower doses for migraine prophylaxis than for their typical antidepressant indications (for example, amitriptyline 10–50 mg vs 100–200 mg for depression). Patients with comorbid conditions such as depression, anxiety, sleep disturbances or other pain disorders may derive dual benefit from the use of tricyclic antidepressants. Because the tricyclics act on various neurotransmitters and receptor systems, side-effects are common. Antimuscarinic side-effects include sedation, dry mouth and cognitive impairment. These drugs are associated with an increased appetite and weight gain and so may best be avoided in patients who are overweight. These drugs can also be associated with cardiac arrhythmia and orthostatic hypotension.

Selective serotonin reuptake inhibitors

In the same meta-analysis, six studies of selective serotonin reuptake inhibitors (SSRIs) that measured effects on headache burden found no significant benefit, and it was suggested that further studies are needed to demonstrate the effectiveness of SSRIs in preventing either migraine or tension-type headaches. The usefulness of these agents for migraine prophylaxis, as suggested by some headache experts, may lie in their activity as antidepressants in patients who suffer from both profound depression and migraine headaches. Generally, doses similar to those used to treat depression are used for migraine prophylaxis.

Potential drug interactions should be considered before placing patients on SSRIs for migraine prophylaxis. The use of SSRIs in conjunction with triptans for acute migraine treatment carries a small risk of serotonin syndrome. A review of the literature revealed 18 cases of potential serotonin syndrome in patients receiving 5-HT$_{1B/1D}$

agonists with an SSRI or lithium. None of the patients had severe symptoms. The symptoms tended to be mild to moderate and to resolve when one or more of the agents was discontinued. Serotonin syndrome generally occurs as a result of combining two or more serotonergic agents or of an overdose of one centrally acting agent. Patients may be considered to have serotonin syndrome when they have at least three of the following: mental status changes, agitation, myoclonus, hyperreflexia, diaphoresis, shivering, tremor, diarrhea, incoordination or fever (with other potential causes excluded).

Non-steroidal anti-inflammatory drugs

These agents are best used for short-term or episodic migraines rather than as long-term prophylaxis in migraineurs. Thus, NSAIDs may be particularly useful in patients who suffer mainly from menstrual or exertional migraine. Unfortunately, if NSAIDs are used as prophylaxis, their acute use may be limited. Side-effects associated with NSAID use are typically gastrointestinal and include nausea, vomiting and gastritis. Patients with migraine headache who also suffer from arthritis or other pain disorders may benefit doubly from NSAID treatment. NSAIDs should not be used by patients who have a history of peptic ulcer disease or gastritis, nor should they be combined with other NSAIDs or aspirin-containing compounds.

Antiepileptic drugs

Antiepileptic drugs may be especially useful in migraineurs who have concomitant epilepsy. They may also be of particular benefit in patients with other comorbidities, such as anxiety, manic-depressive illness, depression, Raynaud's disease or diabetes. To date, only divalproex sodium has received FDA approval for migraine prevention. Double-blind, placebo-controlled studies have found divalproex sodium (valproate) to be substantially more efficacious than placebo in reducing the frequency of migraine attacks as follows.

- A mean 4-week migraine frequency of 3.5 episodes with valproate versus 5.7 with placebo was found in one study, together with a 50% or greater reduction in 4-week migraine frequency over baseline in 48% of patients compared with 14% for placebo.

TABLE 7.3

Migraine prophylactic drugs

Drug	Clinical efficacy	Scientific proof of efficacy	Side-effect potential
Beta-blockers (propranolol, timolol, nadalol, atenolol, metoprolol)	++++	++++	++
Tricyclic antidepressants (amitriptyline)	++++	++++	++
Calcium channel blockers			
– flunarizine	++	+++	+++
– verapamil	+	+	+
Antiepileptics			
– divalproex	++++	+++	+++
– gabapentin	++	++	+++
– topiramate	++	++	+++
NSAIDs	++	+++	++
Serotonin antagonists (methysergide)	+++	++	+++

Adapted, with permission, from Silberstein 2000

- Compared with 21% for placebo, 44% of patients receiving valproate experienced 50% or greater decrease in migraine attack frequencies in another study.

Valproate may prove useful in patients in whom β-blockers are ineffective, not tolerated or contraindicated. Doses lower than those typically used for epilepsy may be given to patients for migraine prevention (500–1000 mg/day). Valproate should not be given to patients who are pregnant or to those with a history of liver disease, pancreatitis or thrombocytopenia. Because of the rare potential for hepatotoxicity with valproate, it is prudent to perform baseline liver function tests. Other side-effects that may occur in patients treated with valproate include polycystic ovary syndrome, weight gain, hair loss, sedation, cognitive changes, tremor, nausea and vomiting. There is a potential for drug interactions with overuse of short-acting barbiturates. Drug interactions may occur with oral contraceptives.

Gabapentin has also been used in migraine prophylaxis. The mechanism of action of this antiepileptic drug in migraine is not known. In the setting of migraine prevention, an open-label study and a placebo-controlled trial have shown gabapentin to be efficacious.

- In the open-label study, gabapentin (600–1800 mg) was associated with a greater than 50% reduction in migraine frequency in 59% of patients. Also substantially decreased on gabapentin were duration of migraine episodes, peak intensity, severity related to functional ability, and the amount of symptomatic medication required. Of patients with transformed migraine included in the study, 48% had a greater than 50% decrease in headache days.

- The placebo-controlled study reported that the percentage of patients with at least a 50% reduction in the frequency of migraine headache was significantly higher in the 2400 mg/day gabapentin group than in the placebo group: 46% versus 16%. The agent was well tolerated, with only minor adverse events reported – somnolence and dizziness. Only 8% of patients withdrew from the study due to side-effects from gabapentin, compared with 2% treated with placebo.

As with divalproex sodium, gabapentin should not be given to pregnant patients.

Topiramate is an antiepileptic agent that has shown some promise in the prevention of migraine, on the basis of two small double-blind placebo-controlled studies. Like other anticonvulsants, lower dosages of topiramate (75–150 mg/day) are used in migraine prophylaxis than in the treatment of seizure disorders. Side-effects associated with topiramate include paresthesias, weight loss, anorexia, altered taste and memory impairment. There have been several reports of serious liver toxicity and acute angle closure glaucoma in patients receiving topiramate, although a definite causal relationship has not yet been demonstrated. Because of its tendency to cause weight loss, topiramate may provide extra benefit to obese or overweight patients. As with the other antiepileptic agents discussed, topiramate is contraindicated in pregnancy.

Other agents

A variety of other types of agents have been used in migraine prophylaxis. These include riboflavin, magnesium and botulinum toxin. A double-blind, placebo-controlled trial of riboflavin, 400 mg/day, found that the agent reduced migraine attack frequency by 50% or more in 56% of patients compared with 19% of placebo patients. Adverse events associated with riboflavin were minor and included diarrhea and polyuria. These results with riboflavin have not been replicated in clinical practice; thus, riboflavin, used in isolation, has not seen widespread use in migraine prophylaxis.

Magnesium has been proposed to play a role in migraine pathogenesis based on its modulatory role on NMDA receptor responsiveness to glutamate. Glutamate-induced NMDA receptor activation is involved in cortical spreading depression, the presumed pathophysiological substrate of the migraine aura (Chapter 4). To date, magnesium replacement has been studied in two controlled trials of migraine prevention and in one trial of migraine associated with the premenstrual syndrome. Two of the three studies favored the use of magnesium over placebo, while the third study failed to show any added benefit. Because of its favorable safety and tolerability profile, oral magnesium may also be used as adjunctive therapy with other conventional preventive therapies.

Botulinum toxin has been suggested as being potentially useful for migraine prophylaxis. Injection of 25 units of botulinum toxin was shown to significantly reduce the frequency and severity of migraine attacks as well as the use of acute medication and migraine-associated vomiting. Botulinum toxin may produce excessive or adjacent muscle weakness and pain in the injection area. Patients with disorders involving the neuromuscular junction or those who take agents that interfere with neuromuscular transmission are not good candidates for botulinum toxin. Further study is needed to determine whether this agent will be beneficial as preventive therapy in migraine sufferers.

Other agents that have generated interest from open-label experience for migraine prophylaxis include leukotriene antagonists such as montelukast, the selective serotonin and norepinephrine reuptake inhibitor venlafaxine, nefazodone, and the antiepileptic medications tiagabine and levetiracetam. Controlled studies with these agents need to be conducted in migraine patients to evaluate their potential activity in preventing migraine.

Combined prophylactic treatment

Patients with refractory headache unresponsive to monotherapy may benefit from combination therapy with more than one prophylactic agent. The patient's specific comorbidities will determine the appropriate combination of agents. Certain combinations, such as β-blockers and calcium channel antagonists, are best avoided or may be contraindicated. Whenever agents are combined, one should keep in mind the possibility of increased side-effects that may have a negative impact on adherence to therapy. On the other hand, two medications with different mechanisms of action may potentiate the effect of each and may be able to be used in lower dosages, thereby minimizing the side-effects of increasing the dosage of one of them to a high level.

Prophylactic treatment – Key points

- Prophylactic therapy should be considered in patients with frequent attacks, and in those responding poorly to optimal analgesic therapy.
- Beta-blockers (propranolol or atenolol) and pizotifen (when available) are agents of first choice.
- Tricyclic antidepressants, valproate, methysergide and regular non-steroidal anti-inflammatory drugs are also of proven value.

Key references

Bendtsen L, Jensen R, Olesen J. A non-selective (amitriptyline), but not a selective (citalopram), serotonin reuptake inhibitor is effective in the prophylactic treatment of chronic tension-type headache. *J Neurol Neurosurg Psychiatry* 1996;61:285–90.

Bosanquet N, Zammit-Lucia J. Migraine: prevention or cure? *Br J Med Econ* 1992;2:81–91.

Diener HC. Flunarizine for migraine prophylaxis. In: Diener HC, ed. Drug Treatment of Migraine and Other Headaches. *Monogr Clin Neurosci*. Basel: Karger, 2000;17:269–78.

Gardner DM, Lynd LD. Sumatriptan contraindications and the serotonin syndrome. *Ann Pharmacother* 1998;32:33–8.

Holroyd KA, Penzien DB, Cordingly GE. Propranolol in the management of recurrent migraine: a meta-analytic review. *Headache* 1991;31:333–40.

Klapper J for the Divalproex Sodium in Migraine Prophylaxis Study Group. Divalproex sodium in migraine prophylaxis: a dose-controlled study. *Cephalalgia* 1997;17:103–8.

Mathew NT, Saper JR, Silberstein SD et al. Migraine prophylaxis with divalproex. *Arch Neurol* 1995;52:281–6.

Mathew NT, Rapoport A, Saper J et al. Efficacy of gabapentin in migraine prophylaxis. *Headache* 2001;41(2):119–28.

Migraine–Nimopidine European Study Group (MINES). European multicenter trial of nimodipine in the prophylaxis of common migraine (migraine without aura). *Headache* 1989;29:633–8.

Schoenen J, Jacquy J, Lenaerts M. Effectiveness of high-dose riboflavin in migraine prophylaxis. A randomized controlled trial. *Neurology* 1998;50:466–70.

Silberstein SD. Divalproex sodium in headache: literature review and clinical guidelines. *Headache* 1996;36:547–55.

Silberstein SD. Practice parameter: evidence based guidelines for migraine headache (an evidence based review). *Neurology* 2000;55:754–63.

Silberstein SD, Mathew NT, Saper J et al. Botulinum toxin type A as a migraine preventive treatment. *Headache* 2000;40:445–50.

Storey JR, Calder CS, Hart DE, Potter DL. Topiramate in migraine prevention: a double-blind, placebo-controlled study. *Headache* 2001;41:968–75.

Tomkins GE, Jackson JL, O'Malley PG et al. Treatment of chronic headaches with antidepressants: a meta-analysis. *Am J Med* 2001;111:54–63.

Turner P. Which ancillary properties
of beta-adrenoceptor blocking drugs
influence their therapeutic or adverse
effects? A review. *J R Soc Med*
1991;84:672–4.

Chronic daily headache (CDH) is arbitrarily defined as headaches which occur more often than 15 days per month or 180 days per year. After the exclusion of secondary causes, CDH can be divided into two primary groups based on the duration of individual headache episodes (Table 8.1). Although a classification of CDH does not yet exist, there is an emerging consensus based on the clinical features of these disorders (Table 8.2), and a modified version of these criteria is expected to appear in the revised International Headache Society classification criteria in 2003.

Primary CDH occurs in 4–5% of the population. Population-based estimates for the 1-year period prevalence of chronic tension-type headache (CTTH) range from 1.7% to 3%, while 1.3–2.4% meet the proposed criteria for chronic migraine (CM). The epidemiology of CM is similar to that of episodic migraine, with a 2.4:1 female

TABLE 8.1

Classification of primary chronic daily headache

Duration > 4 hours

- Chronic migraine ('transformed migraine')
- Chronic tension-type headache
- New daily persistent headache
- Hemicrania continua

Duration ≤ 4 hours

- Cluster headache
- Paroxysmal hemicranias
- Hypnic headache
- SUNCT syndrome

SUNCT, short-lasting unilateral neuralgiform headache attacks with conjunctival injection and tearing

TABLE 8.2

Criteria for types of chronic daily headache

Chronic migraine

- Daily or almost daily (≥ 15 days/month) head pain for ≥ 1 month
- Average headache duration of > 4 hours per day (untreated)
- At least one of:
  - history of episodic migraine (IHS)
- – history of increasing headache frequency with decreasing average severity of migrainous features over ≥ 3 months
- – headache at some time meets IHS criteria for migraine other than duration
- No evidence of organic disease

Chronic tension-type headache

- Average frequency > 15 days/month with average duration > 4 hours/day if untreated, for ≥ 3 months
- At least 3 of:
  - pressing/tightening quality
  - mild or moderate (does not prohibit activities)
  - bilateral
  - no aggravation by routine physical activity
- History of ETTH
- Gradual increase (evolution) over ≥ 3 months
- Both of the following:
  - no nausea (anorexia may occur)
  - no photophobia, no phonophobia
- No evidence of organic disease

New daily persistent headache (NDPH)

- Average frequency ≥ 15 days/month for ≥ 1 month
- Average duration > 4 hours (frequently constant but may fluctuate with medication)
- No history of migraine or TTH which increases in frequency and decreases in severity with onset of NDPH
- Acute onset (developing in < 3 days) of constant unremitting headache
- Constant in location
- No evidence of organic disease

ETTH, episodic tension-type headache; IHS, International Headache Society; TTH, tension-type headache preponderance and an inverse relation with educational level. Recently, it has also been demonstrated that there is a 2.1- to 3.9-fold increased risk of CTTH in the parents, siblings and children of CTTH patients.

In specialist headache centers, approximately 35–80% of patients who seek treatment suffer from CDH. Of these, patients with CM constitute the overwhelming majority. In these patient samples, analgesic overuse ranges from 50–82%, while population-based studies have demonstrated analgesic overuse in 31% of patients with CM, compared with 18% in those with CTTH. In the great majority of patients (70–80%), there is a gradual evolution of CDH from an episodic pattern. It is unclear whether analgesic overuse is a cause or consequence of increasingly frequent headaches, but it seems clear that in many patients the excessive use of immediate-relief medications is important in the maintenance and amplification of CDH.

Analgesic overuse/rebound headache

Rebound headache can be defined as the perpetuation or maintenance of chronic head pain in chronic headache sufferers, caused by the frequent and excessive use of immediate relief medications (see Chapter 6). Although medication rebound has not been demonstrated in placebo-controlled trials, withdrawal headache has been shown in a controlled trial of caffeine withdrawal, and caffeine-containing medications are frequently implicated in CDH with analgesic overuse. Although rebound is believed to occur with simple and combination analgesics as well as opioids, especially those containing caffeine and butalbital, migraine-specific drugs such as ergotamine tartrate and the triptans can also induce a rebound headache phenomenon. The actual dosage limits and the time needed to develop rebound headaches have not been defined in rigorous studies. However, it is generally believed that overuse of medication may be responsible for the maintenance of a chronic daily headache pattern when patients take:

- 3 or more simple analgesics per day on 5 or more days per week
- 1 or more triptan or combination analgesic (containing butalbital, caffeine or sedative) on 3 or more days per week
- 1 or more opiate or ergotamine tartrate dose on 2 or more days per week.

The fact that the mere discontinuation of these medications results in significant improvement in headache is perhaps the most convincing evidence for the existence of analgesic, ergotamine and triptan rebound headache. Overuse of acute medications may be responsible in part for the transformation of episodic migraine or tension-type headache into a chronic daily pattern; however, some patients develop CM or CTTH without overusing medication, while others continue to have daily headaches despite the discontinuation of immediate relief medication.

Treatment of patients with CDH who take excessive amounts of immediate relief medication must entail tapering or discontinuing the potentially offending medications. Continued overuse is thought to neutralize the effectiveness of prophylactic medications, and prolonged use of large amounts of medication may cause renal or hepatic toxicity in addition to tolerance, habituation or dependence.

Psychiatric comorbidity

Psychiatric comorbidity may occur in up to 90% of patients with CDH. Generalized anxiety has been demonstrated in 70%, and major depression may occur in at least 25% of patients. Psychiatric comorbidity may also be an indicator of those patients who may be refractory to medical therapy. CDH patients who have major depression or abnormal Beck Depression Inventory scores have worse outcomes at 3–6 months compared with patients who are not depressed. Abnormal Minnesota Multiphasic Personality Inventory, physical, emotional or sexual abuse, and a positive dexamethasone suppression test also correlate with a poor response to aggressive management. Appropriate evaluation and management of psychiatric comorbidity is therefore important to optimize the likelihood of a favorable outcome.

Pathogenesis

The pathogenesis of CDH is unknown. However, neurophysiologic and neuroimaging findings indicate a number of possible explanations, including sensitization (chronic activation) of peripheral and central trigeminal pain-sensitive neurons and defective pain modulation due to dysfunctional central antinociception. Recent imaging data provide the most specific evidence of disturbed function of the periaqueductal gray (PAG) in patients with migraine. The PAG is the center of a powerful descending antinociceptive neuronal network and considered a major nodal point in the central nervous system, regulating autonomic adjustments to antinociceptive, autonomic and behavioral responses to threat. In these studies, iron levels (a marker of disturbed neuronal function) were equally elevated in the PAG of subjects with migraine with or without aura. Not only was a significant increase in tissue non-heme iron found in patients with episodic and chronic migraine compared with controls, but levels increased with the duration of illness. Because there was no correlation with age in any group, these data suggest that iron accumulation over time in the episodic and chronic migraine groups may be caused by repeated headache attacks.

Management

In patients with primary CDH, it is important to identify the subtype of CDH and evaluate for the presence of analgesic overuse and psychiatric comorbidity. A combination of pharmacological and behavioral interventions is usually necessary for a favorable outcome. The essential features of an effective treatment regimen include the following.

- Give adequate instruction about the biology of CDH, the frequent occurrence of depression and anxiety which needs to be addressed, and the self-sustaining and deleterious effects of certain medications used in excessive and frequent quantities.
- Discontinue all potentially offending medications by outpatient or inpatient detoxification. Some authorities feel that tapering is often necessary for patients on large dosages of opiates or butalbital-containing analgesics.
- Initiate preventive therapy – options include amitriptyline, divalproex, topiramate, tizanidine, Cox-2 inhibitors and botulinum toxin.
- Limit symptomatic medication to moderate or severe breakthrough headaches and to the following medications:
  - long-acting NSAIDS
  - dihydroergotamine (DHE-45)
  - triptans (if not one of the offending medications and ≤ 2 dosages per week)

- Apply behavioral intervention:
  - biofeedback and relaxation therapy
  - cognitive behavioral therapy
  - individual/family counseling
  - dietary instructions
  - physical exercise / physical therapy (where appropriate)
  - expectations and follow-up plan – patients who overuse acute medication may not become fully responsive to acute and preventive treatment for 3–8 weeks after overuse is eliminated.

Admission to hospital may be necessary for those who fail outpatient treatment or consume large quantities of opioids or butalbital-containing analgesics, as well as those with significant psychological, behavioral or medical comorbidities. A variety of medications are used intravenously in the inpatient setting in an attempt to terminate the daily cycle of headache, while overused medications are being tapered or discontinued and preventive therapies are being initiated. Inpatient stay usually lasts 2–3 days and involves the repetitive administration of one or more agents such as dihydroergotamine, divalproex sodium, a dopamine antagonist (prochlorperazine, droperidol) or corticosteroids.

Prognosis

The natural history of untreated primary CDH and rebound headache will likely never be known because of the ethical considerations involved. There are no literature reports of spontaneous improvement of rebound headache, although this may happen. A variety of studies have, however, evaluated the long-term outcome in cohorts of patients with CDH with and without rebound. Overall, on the basis of recent studies with 2–4 year follow-up of patients with CDH with analgesic overuse, it appears that approximately two-thirds of patients continue to have persistent headache after appropriate management. A significant proportion of these patients return to overusing immediate-relief medications. These rather disturbing data underscore the importance of early and aggressive acute and preventive treatment in those patients whose attacks begin to escalate in frequency, and highlights the need for prospective studies designed to identify the patient characteristics which may be predictive of progression to chronic daily headache. A better understanding of the pathophysiology of this progression will, one hopes, lead to improved therapies.

Chronic daily headache – Key points

- Patients with more than 15 days of headache each month are considered to have chronic daily headache (CDH).
- Four to five percent of the population have incessant headaches; about half of these used to have migraine and half episodic tension-type headache.
- Most patients seeking advice for CDH are overusing analgesics, and some respond to reassurance, supportive therapy, withdrawal of offending medications, and substitution with tricyclic antidepressants and non-steroidal anti-inflammatory drugs.

Key references

Bendtsen L. Central sensitization in tension-type headache – possible pathophysiologic mechanisms. *Cephalalgia* 2002;20:486–508.

Castillo J, Munoz P, Guitera V, Pasqual J. Epidemiology of chronic daily headache in the general population. *Headache* 1999;39:190–6.

Mathew NT. Transformed or evolutional migraine. *Headache* 1987;27:305–6.

Mathew NT, Kurman R, Perez F. Drug induced refractory headache – clinical features and management. *Headache* 1990;30:634–8.

Scher AI, Stewart WF, Liberman J, Lipton RB. Prevalence of frequent headache in a population sample. *Headache* 1998;38:497–506.

Silberstein SD, Lipton RB. Chronic daily headache. *Curr Opin Neurol* 2000;13:277–83.

Silberstein SD, Lipton RB, Sliwinski M. Classification of daily and near daily headaches: field trial of revised IHS criteria. *Neurology* 1996;47:871–5.

Solomon S, Lipton RB, Newman LC. Clinical features of chronic daily headache. *Headache* 1992;32:325–9.

Srikiatkhachorn A, Naovarut T, Govitrapong P. Effect of chronic analgesic exposure on the central serotonin system: a possible mechanism of analgesic abuse headache. *Headache* 2000;40: 343–50.

Wang SJ, Fuh JL, Lu SR et al. Chronic daily headache in Chinese elderly: prevalence, risk factors and biannual follow-up. *Neurology* 2000;54:314–19.

Welch KMA, Nagesh L, Aurora SK, Gelman N. Periaqueductal gray matter dysfunction in migraine: cause or the burden of illness? *Headache* 2001;41:629–37.

Zed PJ, Loewen PS, Robinson G. Medication-induced headache: overview and systematic review of therapeutic approaches. *Ann Pharmacother* 1999;33:61–72.

Cluster headache is perhaps the most easily defined of the primary headache syndromes. The term 'cluster headache' was introduced by Kunkle and his colleagues in 1952 and has now superseded 'periodic migrainous neuralgia'. Cluster headache affects only 5/100 000 population, but these individuals constitute about 10% of the patients seen in a typical migraine clinic. Unlike migraine, which is three times as common in women as in men, the prevalence of cluster headache is about three times higher in men than in women.

Clinical features

Typical cases of cluster headache have a characteristic pattern of symptoms. However, most family physicians see few patients with the condition, and many cases are misdiagnosed and sometimes inappropriately treated before the correct diagnosis is made. Patients experience attacks of extremely severe pain, usually felt in, behind or around one eye, though pains can be felt in the temple, forehead, cheek or jaw, or even in the neck or hemicranially. The pain is always unilateral and repeated attacks nearly always affect the same side. It typically lasts for 60 minutes, and the IHS definition requires that it lasts for under 3 hours. Cluster headache usually involves prolonged, steady pain which has a longer duration than trigeminal neuralgia and does not throb like many cases of migraine. The pain is so severe that patients are unable to lie down, and they characteristically get out of bed and pace about.

Attacks are often accompanied by one or more cranial autonomic symptoms, such as the following.
- The eye can become bloodshot.
- The eye can water profusely.
- The nostril can become blocked or stream.

During the attacks, a few patients develop an overt Horner's syndrome, which can sometimes persist. Although migrainous symptoms are generally less prominent than seen in migraine, nausea, photophobia and phonophobia, and even premonitory symptoms – visual, sensory and motor aura – have been described.

Attacks typically occur one to four times a day, although some patients have as many as eight attacks in a 24-hour period. They often take place at exactly the same times of day, and it is common for patients to wake with a headache about 1–2 hours after falling asleep. Around 90% of patients with cluster headache experience bouts of daily attacks lasting for 4–12 weeks, occurring between twice a year and once every 5 years. Approximately 10% have unremittant daily attacks for periods exceeding 12 months, and often for much longer periods. The long-term follow up of patients with cluster headache has shown that the pattern tends to persist for many years, and remissions, although they may increase in duration, are less common than in migraine.

In most cases, cluster headache starts in the 20s or 30s, perhaps a little later than the onset of typical migraine. There is an excess of smokers among people with cluster headache, but the attacks are the same in non-smokers and the natural history of the condition is not affected if smoking is stopped. Recent evidence indicates that cluster headache can be inherited, possibly as an autosomal-dominant trait in some patients.

Differential diagnosis

Although the history of a cluster headache is often unmistakable, various other possibilities should be considered in the differential diagnosis. Migraine may present with recurrent unilateral headache even with ipsilateral autonomic symptoms, particularly during severe attacks. However, the periodicity of cluster headache is often very stereotyped for a given patient, and the attacks of cluster headache are short-lived (45–90 minutes) compared with those of migraine (4–72 hours). Furthermore, cluster attacks are almost always unilateral, frequently nocturnal, can occur several times per day, and usually are not associated with aura, nausea or vomiting.

Trigeminal neuralgia (see Chapter 1) is characterized by paroxysmal shock-like electric jabs of unilateral pain, most commonly limited to the distribution of the second and/or third divisions of the trigeminal nerve, and rarely confined to the periorbital region. The pain can be triggered by stimulation of limited areas of facial skin or oral mucosa. Other disorders to be considered are dissection of the cervicocephalic cerebral blood vessels (carotid or vertebral), sinusitis, glaucoma, intracranial aneurysms, tumors or arteriovenous malformations, and even cervical cord lesions (meningioma) or infarction. In many of these instances, however, the history lacks the typical stereotyped periodicity of attack and remission phases, there are abnormalities on examination, or the response to conventional medications is lacking.

Finally, there are a number of primary headache syndromes which may closely resemble cluster headache, such as chronic and episodic paroxysmal hemicrania, SUNCT syndrome, and hemicrania continua (Table 9.1). Collectively, these disorders are referred to as 'trigeminal-autonomic cephalgias' because of the trigeminal distribution of pain and the associated autonomic signs. They are characterized by discrete short-lasting episodic attacks of intense unilateral orbital-temporal headache associated with robust ipsilateral autonomic signs. These syndromes may be associated with nocturnal attacks. Cluster headache and SUNCT syndrome appear to be the only headache disorders that predominate in males. SUNCT syndrome clinically resembles trigeminal neuralgia (brief lancinating pain) except that the paroxysms are slightly longer in duration (30–120 seconds), often confined to or maximal in the periorbital (V1) distribution, and autonomic symptoms and signs are often dramatic.

Compared with cluster headache, these disorders differ mainly in the higher frequency and shorter duration of individual attacks. There is an almost inverse relationship across these disorders: as attack frequency increases, attack duration tends to decrease (Table 9.1). The distinction between cluster headache and other paroxysmal hemicranias is important because of the differential response to therapy. The paroxysmal hemicranias and hemicrania continua often respond in a dramatic fashion to indomethacin, whereas patients with SUNCT syndrome derive no benefit from indomethacin or drugs typically used to treat cluster headache. Some patients with SUNCT syndrome have been reported to respond to carbamazepine, lamotrigine, gabapentin or topiramate.

TABLE 9.1

Cluster headache: comparison with other trigeminal-autonomic cephalgias

	Cluster headache	Chronic paroxysmal hemicrania
Gender (M:F)	3:1	1:3
Attack duration Range Mean	15–180 min 60 min	2–45 min 15 min
Attack frequency	1–3/day Rarely up to 8	1–40/day Usually over 5
Autonomic features	++	++
Indomethacin effect	+/–	++

SUNCT, short-lasting unilateral neuralgiform pain with conjunctival injection and tearing

Pathogenesis

A unifying pathophysiological explanation of cluster headache is not yet available. Any hypothesis must account for the three major features of the syndrome: the trigeminal distribution of pain; the ipsilateral autonomic features; and the tendency for attacks to cluster with striking circadian and circannual consistency.

Three conclusions can be drawn. First, because the pain of cluster headache (CH) is invariably centered on the eye and forehead, activation of trigeminal nociceptive pathways is involved. Second, the ipsilateral autonomic features indicate activation of the cranial parasympathetic system (lacrimation and rhinorrhea) and the ipsilateral sympathetic nerves (ptosis and miosis). In humans, evidence for activation of the trigeminovascular system in cluster headache has been highlighted by a marked increase in the level of calcitonin gene-related peptide (a trigeminal neuropeptide) in the cranial venous circulation during attacks of cluster headache and chronic paroxysmal hemicrania. In addition, evidence of parasympathetic activation in

Episodic paroxysmal hemicrania	SUNCT	Hemicrania continua
1:1	3:1	1:2
1–30 min 15 min	5–250 sec 60 sec	Continuous unilateral headache with
3–30/day Usually over 5	1/day–30/hour Usually over 5/day	exacerbations lasting hours to days
++	++	+
++	–	++

humans has been corroborated by the finding of significantly elevated levels of vasoactive intestinal polypeptide (a parasympathetic neuropeptide) during attacks of CH where ipsilateral autonomic features are robust.

The cavernous carotid artery has been suggested as a likely site of involvement since it is here that the trigeminal, parasympathetic and sympathetic fibers converge. Recently, PET studies during precipitated attacks of CH have also demonstrated bilateral activation (more marked on the side of the headache) in the region of the cavernous sinus, thought to be indicative of increased flow in the cavernous portion of the internal carotid arteries. However, the same pattern of activation using PET has also been shown in migraine as well as in healthy controls with experimentally induced first-division trigeminal pain elicited with capsaicin. Despite the theory that an inflammatory process in the cavernous sinus and tributary veins may be the underlying mechanism of cluster headache, an MRI study of cluster patients revealed no definite pathological changes in this region.

Orbital phlebography studies, which have demonstrated venous outflow obstruction in the region of the cavernous sinus, are not specific to cluster headache and have been demonstrated in patients with Tolosa Hunt syndrome, hemicrania continua, SUNCT syndrome, chronic paroxysmal hemicrania, cervicogenic headache, migraine and tension-type headache. These data strongly suggest that the flow changes seen during CH attacks are an epiphenomenon of trigeminal activation and do not play a causal role in the genesis of CH. These findings support the concept of cluster headache as a neurovascular syndrome rather than simply a 'vascular headache' disorder.

Finally, the remarkable and often clockwork consistency and seasonal predilection of attacks strongly suggests that a disturbance exists in the biological clock or pacemaker, which in humans is located in the hypothalamic gray in an area known as the suprachiasmatic nucleus. Substantially lowered concentrations of plasma testosterone during the cluster headache period in men provided the first evidence of hypothalamic involvement in cluster headache pathogenesis. This finding was followed by reports of alterations in the production of a wide range of secretory circadian rhythms involving luteinizing hormone (LH), cortisol, melatonin and prolactin (PRL), as well as altered responses in the production of cortisol, LH, follicle-stimulating hormone, PRL, growth hormone and thyroid-stimulating hormone to diverse challenges in cluster headache.

The most direct and convincing evidence for the role of the hypothalamus in cluster headache pathogenesis has come from functional and morphometric neuroimaging. Marked functional activation has been demonstrated, by PET imaging, in the ipsilateral ventral hypothalamic gray matter during attacks of acute CH induced by nitroglycerin. This finding appears to be specific for CH and perhaps other related trigeminal autonomic cephalgias, as the same pattern of activation in this region of the hypothalamus was recently demonstrated in a patient with SUNCT syndrome. This pattern of activation has not been seen during attacks of migraine or experimentally induced ophthalmic (first-division) pain induced by capsaicin injection into the forehead of control subjects.

Management

Acute. Because of the rapid onset and short time to peak intensity of the pain of cluster headache, a fast-acting symptomatic therapy is imperative. Oxygen and subcutaneous sumatriptan provide the most rapid, effective and reliable relief for attacks of cluster headache. Oxygen inhalation has been the standard of care for the symptomatic relief of CH since it was introduced as an effective therapy in the 1950s, supported by a double-blind comparison with compressed air in 1985. If delivered at the onset of an attack via a non-rebreathing facial mask at a flow rate of 7 liters per minute for 15 minutes, approximately 70% of patients will obtain relief within 15 minutes. In some patients, oxygen is most effective if taken when the pain is at maximal intensity, whereas in others the attack is delayed for minutes to hours rather than completely aborted. Oxygen therapy has obvious practical limitations in that treatment is not always readily available, and although small portable cylinders are available for use at work or when out of the house, some patients find this to be cumbersome and inconvenient.

Subcutaneous sumatriptan is the most effective self-administered medication for the symptomatic relief of cluster headache. In a placebo-controlled study, 6 mg of sumatriptan delivered subcutaneously was significantly more effective than placebo, with 74% of patients having complete relief by 15 minutes compared with 26% treated with placebo. In long-term open-label studies, sumatriptan is effective in 76–100% of attacks within 15 minutes, with no evidence of tachyphylaxis or rebound even after repetitive daily use for several months. However, sumatriptan is not effective when used before an expected attack in an attempt to prevent the attack, nor is it useful as a prophylactic agent. Although generally well tolerated, sumatriptan is contraindicated in patients with ischemic heart disease, variant angina, cerebrovascular and peripheral vascular disease and uncontrolled hypertension. In this sense, caution must be exercised in patients with CH since the disorder predominates in middle-aged males, often with risk factors for cardiovascular disease, particularly tobacco abuse, which is present in up to 90% of cluster headache sufferers.

Preventive. The importance of an effective preventive regimen during cluster periods cannot be overstated. During cluster periods, individual cluster attacks often occur daily for several weeks to months. Many patients have more than one attack per day (up to eight), and the attacks are severe, short-lived and peak rapidly, making repeated attempts at abortive therapy an exhausting exercise. Furthermore, abortive therapies may be contraindicated, ineffective, not tolerated, or they may merely delay the attack. Treating frequent daily attacks may result in overmedication or toxicity, and finally, repeated attacks of severe pain may unnecessarily prolong suffering.

The primary goals of preventive therapy are to produce a rapid suppression of attacks and to maintain that remission over the expected duration of the cluster period. Secondary objectives are to reduce the headache frequency, as well as attack severity and duration. To achieve these primary goals, preventive therapy can best be thought of in terms of transitional and maintenance prophylaxis. Transitional agents, such as prednisone, induce a rapid suppression of attacks during the time required for the longer-acting maintenance prophylactic agents to take effect, since the maximum benefit from other preventive drugs may not be realized until 2 weeks after treatment is begun. Prednisone may be started at a dosage of 40–60 mg per day and tapered by 10 mg decrements every 2–3 days. Verapamil is the drug of first choice for maintenance prophylaxis. The effective dosage ranges between 240 and 720 mg/day. Lithium (800–1200 mg) and methysergide (4–12 mg) may also be of value and have been used for decades in treating patients with cluster headache. Recently, several anticonvulsants, including divalproex sodium (1000 mg), topiramate (100–200 mg), and gabapentin (900–1200 mg), have emerged as effective preventive treatments for episodic and chronic cluster headache in some patients. In some patients who do not respond optimally to monotherapy, a combination of preventive drugs may prove useful.

Surgery. Occasionally, patients with intractable chronic cluster headache, particularly if it remains strictly unilateral, may warrant surgical treatment. Radiofrequency thermocoagulation of the trigeminal ganglion, as for trigeminal neuralgia, is the most commonly used technique, though the ophthalmic division of the ganglion should be lesioned, and control of cluster headache requires powerful thermocoagulation which is likely to leave the patient with some permanent anesthesia. The role of stimulation of the posterior hypothalamus awaits further safety and efficacy studies.

Cluster headache – Key points

- Cluster headache is a rare but often devastating pain, commoner in men.
- Sufferers typically have 1–4 severe unilateral pains daily, lasting less than 3 hours.
- There are often autonomic symptoms, such as a ptosis, a watering or bloodshot eye, and blocked or watering nose.
- Most patients have their pain in bouts, lasting 4–12 weeks, every 6 months to 5 years.
- For analgesia, 100% oxygen and parenteral sumatriptan are the most effective.
- Prophylaxis is preferable, with verapamil, corticosteroids, lithium carbonate or gabapentin.

Key references

Antonaci F, Sjaastad O. Chronic paroxysmal hemicrania (CPH): a review of the clinical manifestations. *Headache* 1989;29:648–56.

Dodick D, Rozen TC, Goadsby PJ, Silberstein SD. Cluster headache. *Cephalalgia* 2000;20:787–803.

Ekbom K. Treatment of cluster headache: clinical trials, design and results. *Cephalalgia* 1995(suppl 15): 33–6.

Gobel H, Lindner V, Pfaffenrath V et al. Acute therapy of episodic and chronic cluster headache with sumatriptan s.c. Results of a one-year long-term study. *Nervenarzt* 1998;69:320–9.

Goadsby PJ, Lipton RB. A review of paroxysmal hemicranias, SUNCT syndrome and other short-lasting headaches with autonomic features, including new cases. *Brain* 1997;120:193–209.

Kunkle EC, Pfeiffer J, Wilhoit WM et al. Recurrent brief headache in 'cluster' pattern. *Trans Am Neurol Assoc* 1952;77:240–3.

Leone M, Franzini A, Bussone G. Stereotactic stimulation of posterior hypothalamic gray matter in a patient with intractable cluster headache. *N Engl J Med* 2001;345:1428–9.

May A, Bahra A, Buchel C et al. Hypothalamic activation in cluster headache attacks. *Lancet* 1998;352:275–78.

Onofrio BM, Campbell JK. Surgical treatment of chronic cluster headache. *Mayo Clin Proc* 1986;61:537–44.

Russell MB, Andersson PG, Iselius L. Cluster headache is an inherited disorder in some families. *Headache* 1996;36:608–12.

The Subcutaneous Sumatriptan International Study Group. Treatment of acute cluster headache with sumatriptan. *N Engl J Med* 1991;325:322–6.

Headache is common immediately after significant head injuries, particularly if there have been complications, such as subarachnoid hemorrhage, intracranial or subdural hematomas, or meningitis. Even after exclusion of these conditions, chronic persistent headache is the most common symptom to follow head injury, occurring in 40–70% of patients in prospective surveys. A large study undertaken in Newcastle, UK, suggested that in 50% of these patients the headache resolved within 1 week, and in two-thirds by 6–8 weeks. However, others may experience headache for 1–2 years after the head injury.

There is only an imperfect correlation of the headache with the severity of the injury as judged by the duration of post-traumatic amnesia. The incidence of headache is lowest after recreational accidents and highest after injuries occurring at work. In the Newcastle series, 12% of patients were found to have headache 6 months after the injury, that was not present at the time of discharge from hospital. These patients were significantly more likely to be depressed, and were often pursuing compensation claims.

Post-traumatic headache is usually intermittent, though episodes can last from minutes to days. It can be generalized or localized, and steady or throbbing. It is often made worse by postural change or effort.

Mechanisms

The mechanisms of post-traumatic headache are poorly understood. Most affected patients also have significant neck injury, which may not involve actual bony fracture. Soft tissue injuries to the neck can interfere with upper cervical nerve roots running onto the scalp, as well as producing secondary neck spasm which can also radiate up onto the head. In other patients, discomfort may come from damage to small nerves in the scalp as a direct result of a laceration. Head injuries may cause damage to pain-sensitive structures within the head, such as large arteries and veins. Shearing of individual nerve fibers may also make a contribution. There is little doubt that depression plays a major role in post-traumatic headache, particularly in those who have no headache at the time of discharge from hospital.

Post-traumatic migraine

It has been recognized since the pioneering reports of Matthews that relatively trivial head injuries can trigger single migraine-like episodes, often including a visual or sensory aura as well as localized headache, nausea and vomiting, starting 1–10 minutes after the impact. Originally described in footballers, this condition occurs in individuals undertaking a variety of contact sports. A similar mechanism is probably responsible for transient acute hemiplegias following head injuries in children, which often occur in the absence of an overt CT scan abnormality. Direct cortical injury (particularly if the skull is relatively deformable) probably triggers spreading depression akin to the supposed mechanism of spontaneous migraine. Attacks resolve spontaneously and little treatment is usually required, though recurrent episodes may curtail the career of a professional footballer.

Whether recurrent attacks of typical migraine can be triggered by a single head injury remains controversial. Head injuries are common in adolescents and young adults – people at the age migraine attacks are likely to start. Studies of several large series of patients with head injury failed to show an increase in the frequency of migrainous attacks after the accident. However, a recent study of 29 individuals in Copenhagen showed that patients with post-traumatic migraine were less likely to have a family history of migraine than those whose migraine did not date from a head injury. This suggests that there may be a causative relationship between head injury and the subsequent onset of migraine.

Management

The management of post-traumatic headache has always been difficult. After investigation, if necessary, to exclude a structural abnormality, the patient should be reassured that even the most persistent headache usually fades 1–3 years after the original injury. The view that persistence was linked to compensation claims has now been discredited, at least for early-onset headache; indeed, the headache often outlasts the legal settlement. The suggestion that many people with post-traumatic headache become depressed, particularly if they developed the condition some time after the injury, has led to the widespread use of antidepressant therapy. However, few properly controlled studies have been carried out to confirm this. Most of these patients are best managed with mild analgesics, particularly NSAIDs, with psychological support and counseling when necessary. Pain originating from the neck may be best managed with a temporary cervical collar, the injection of local anesthetic to tender spots, or physiotherapy.

Post-traumatic headache – Key points

- Headache follows head injury in 40–70% of victims.
- The risk is imperfectly related to the severity of the injury.
- Delayed headache is often due to depression.
- Neck and scalp injury may be responsible.
- In most cases the pain resolves within a few weeks, but some patients may experience headache for 1–2 years after the injury.
- Patients are best managed with tricyclic antidepressants and non-steroidal anti-inflammatory drugs.

Key references

Cartlidge NEF, Shaw DA, Kalbag RM. Head injury. In: *Major Problems in Neurology*. London: WB Saunders, 1981.

Haas DC, Lourie H. Trauma-triggered migraine: an explanation for common neurological attacks after mild head injury. *J Neurosurg* 1988;68:181–8.

Matthews WB. Footballer's migraine. *BMJ* 1972;2:326–7.

Russell MB, Olesen J. Migraine associated with head trauma. *Cephalalgia* 1996;16:375.

Solomon, S. Posttraumatic migraine. *Headache* 1998;38:772–8.

Recognition of morbidity

More recent epidemiological surveys using the IHS criteria confirm the amount of time lost from and reduced efficacy at work. Such evidence of the overall cost of migraine in the community would help to increase the resources made available, both for treatment and for research into new medication.

Genetics

The precise molecular mechanism of the subtype of familial hemiplegic migraine linked to chromosome 19 is already being elucidated, and the same should apply to markers for the other subtypes. Genetic studies of more typical migraine with and without aura are in progress in several centers, and it may be possible to correlate not only the patients' symptoms but also the response to different types of medication to particular genetic abnormalities.

Triptans

There are now seven triptans available for the treatment of migraine. They have unquestionably advanced the treatment of migraine. A greater understanding of the pharmacology of this group of drugs and particularly their role in suppressing pain pathways within the central nervous system may lead to the development of more selective agents without the liability associated with vasoconstriction.

Other acute treatments

Antagonists of substance P have proved disappointing. It remains possible that, in studies, inhibitors of other mediators (such as peptides, e.g. CGRP) will prove efficacious. Other molecular targets for acute therapy have been identified – neuronal 5-HT, NMDA and adenosine receptors, NOS inhibitors – and drug discovery programs are currently underway. As has long been the case with migraine, we are likely to learn more about the pharmacology of the disease from these studies than we can predict in the opposite direction.

Prophylactic therapy

Progress in the development of new selective prophylactic treatments has disappointingly lagged behind developments in acute treatment. This area is a major priority for the future.

Analgesic rebound headache

The publicity that has been given to this condition in recent years has probably done more to help patients with chronic headache than any other single maneuver (see Chapter 8).

Useful addresses

American Council for Headache
Education (ACHE)
19 Mantua Road,
Mt Royal, NJ 08061, USA
phone 856 423 0258
fax 856 423 0082
achehq@talley.com
www.achenet.org

American Headache Society
(formerly the American
Association for the Study of
Headache)
19 Mantua Road,
Mount Royal, NJ 08061, USA
phone 856 423 0043
fax 856 423 0082
ahshq@talley.com
www.ahsnet.org

International Headache Society
Rosemary Chilcott, Permanent
Secretary,
Oakwood, 9 Willowmead Drive,
Prestbury, Cheshire SK10 4BU,
UK
phone +44 (0)1625 828663
fax +44 (0)1625 828494
www.i-h-s.org

Migraine Action Association
(formerly the British Migraine
Association)
Unit 6, Oakley Hay Lodge
Business Park,
Great Folds Road, Great Oakley,
Northants NN18 9AS, UK
phone 01536 461333
fax 01536 461444
www.migraine.org.uk

Migraine Trust
45 Great Ormond Street,
London WC1N 3HZ, UK
phone 020 7831 4818
fax 020 7831 5174
www.migrainetrust.org

National Headache Foundation
428 West St James Place,
Second floor,
Chicago, IL 60614, USA
phone 888 643 5552
www.headaches.org

Organisation for Understanding
Cluster Headaches (OUCH)
OUCH (UK), Registered Office,
94 London Road,
Leicester LE2 0QS, UK
phone 0161 2721702
www.clusterheadaches.org.uk

World Headache Alliance
3288 Old Coach Road,
Burlington, Ontario,
Canada L7N 3P7
info@w-h-a.org
www.w-h-a.org/wha/index.asp

Index